BASIC MEDICAL TERMINOLOGY CONCEPTS

Second Edition

MARILYN WHITE WILSON

BRADY
REGENTS/PRENTICE HALL
Englewood Cliffs, New Jersey 07632

Library of Congress Cataloging-in-Publication Data
Wilson, Marilyn White, 1941–
   Basic medical terminology concepts / Marilyn White Wilson.—2nd ed.
       p. cm.
   Includes index.
   ISBN 0-8359-4956-7 (pbk.)
   1. Medicine—Terminology.   2. Medicine—Terminology—Problems, exercises, etc.
I. Title.
   [DNLM: 1. Nomenclature—problems.   W 18 W7511b 1995]
R123.W48 1995
610'. 14—dc20
DNLM/DLC
for Library of Congress   94-45259
                                                                 CIP

Editorial/production supervision: *Susan Geraghty*
Cover design: *Amy Rosen*
Manufacturing buyer: *Ilene Sanford*
Typesetting and art: *LeGwin Associates*
Printing and binding: *R.R. Donnelley*

 © 1996 by Prentice-Hall, Inc.
A Simon & Schuster Company
Englewood Cliffs, New Jersey 07632

Printed in the United States of America
10 9 8 7 6 5

ISBN 0-8359-4956-7

Prentice-Hall International (UK) Limited, *London*
Prentice-Hall of Australia Pty. Limited, *Sydney*
Prentice-Hall Canada Inc., *Toronto*
Prentice-Hall Hispanoamericana, S.A., *Mexico*
Prentice-Hall of India Private Limited, *New Delhi*
Prentice-Hall of Japan, Inc., *Tokyo*
Simon & Schuster Asia Pte. Ltd., *Singapore*
Editora Prentice-Hall do Brasil, Ltda., *Rio de Janeiro*

DEDICATION

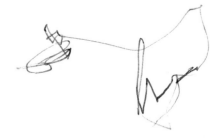

I again express my gratitude to James D. O'Keefe, MD, for his patience those many years ago. Because of the numbers, it is impossible to individually thank the physicians and their staff who have shared information for this revision. Of course, Tamasyn A. Wilson and James F. Wilson get thanks again. Finally, saying thank you is inadequate for the many, many students whose valuable input, comments, and suggestions have made me a better teacher. They are a true treasure.

CONTENTS

PREFACE   ix

INTRODUCTION   1

PRETEST   5

SELF-DEFINING WORDS   13

1   PRONOUNCING AND SPELLING MEDICAL TERMS   15

Consonants   15
Vowels   16
Forming Plurals   17
Spelling Rules   17

2   BODY AND DISEASE SCIENCES   19

Study of the Body   19
Biological Structure and Functions   20
Basic Systems   21
Medical and Surgical Disciplines
   and Specialties/Specialists   25
Exercises
   1. Medical Disciplines Fill in the Blanks Exercise   41
   2. Medical Disciplines, Branches, Terms, and
        Specialties Exercises   44

3. Specialists and Their Specialties Puzzle 48
4. Body and Disease Sciences Multiple Choice Exercise 50

3 **PREVIEWING PREFIXES** **55**

Prefixes with Meaning and Word Example(s) 55
  Locations and Positions 55
  Time 57
  Negation 57
  Numbers, Amounts, and Comparison 57
  Colors 58
  Size 59
  Miscellaneous 59
  Positions and Locations 60
Abdominal Divisions and Regions 61
Basic Surgical Incisions 63
Positions for Surgery and Examination 64
Exercises
  1. Positions and Locations Matching Exercise 67
  2. Prefix Definition Exercise 68
  3. More Prefixes Definition Exercise 71
  4. Prefix Completion Exercise 73
  5. Prefix Puzzle 76
  6. Abdominal Regions and Incisions Puzzle 78
  7. Prefix Multiple Choice Exercise 79

4 **SUFFERING SUFFIXES** **91**

Suffixes with Meaning and Word Example(s) 91
  Diagnostic/Symptomatic Terms 91
  Size Terms 95
  Treatment, Repair, or Surgical Terms 95
  Miscellaneous Terms 96
Exercises
  1. Suffix Definition Exercise 97
  2. Suffix Matching Exercise 103
  3. Suffix Finding and Matching Exercise 104
  4. Suffix Finding and Matching Exercise 105
  5. Suffix Puzzle 106
  6. Suffix Multiple Choice Exercise 108

5   GETTING DOWN TO ROOTS   116

Roots with Meaning and Word Example(s)   116
   Organs or Body Components Shown in the Male
   (andro) Drawing   116
   Organs or Body Components Shown in the Female
   (gyn/e/ec/eco) in the Drawing   118
   Organs or Body Components Not Shown in Drawings   119
   Miscellaneous Roots   120
   Drawing of the Man   121
   Drawing of the Woman   122
Exercises
   1. Internal Organ Matching Exercise   123
   2. Root Multiple Choice Exercise   124
   3. Root Matching Exercise 133
   4. Root Puzzle   134
   5. Root Matching Exercise   135
   6. Root-Internal Organ Puzzle   136
   7. Root Multiple Choice Exercise   138
   8. Root Identification Exercise   146
   9. The Male Internal Organ Exercise   149
   10. The Female Internal Organ Exercise   150

6   PUTTING IT ALL TOGETHER   151

Exercises
   1. Review Definition Exercise   152
   2. Review Definition Exercise   154
   3. Review Definition Exercise   157
   4. Review Definition Exercise   159
   5. Putting it All Together Puzzle   162
   6. Review Completion Exercise   164
   7. Review of Paragraphs—Translating from
      Medical to Lay Terms   168
   8. Review of Paragraphs—Translating from Lay
      to Medical Terms   172

POSTTEST   174

GLOSSARY   181

INDEX   193

PREFACE

Basic Medical Terminology Concepts introduces a system of medical word analysis that applies to the continual learning of new terminology. It covers approximately 380 prefixes, suffixes, and roots or stems, the ABCs of the medical "language," with a heavy emphasis on the application of newly learned "words" in a variety of exercise formats. Some very basic anatomy is covered, as well as an overview of a variety of medical specialties/specialists. The last chapter concentrates on practical, in-context application of learned prefixes, suffixes, and roots or stems through exercises that include excerpts from actual medical reports. On completion of this text/workbook, the student will be familiar with and knowledgeable about basic medical terms and will have learned the tools to dissect words, understand "created" words, and understand new words by breaking them down, applying the word elements already known, and making an educated guess through context of any new word element in the word. This skill is invaluable for anyone working in any medically related area, including (but not limited to) nurses, transcribers, unit secretaries, schedulers, and coding/billing specialists. Through this system of word analysis/breakdown, there is direct application to the continuous updating of medical terminology used in clinical and research medicine.

The particular concept of learning medical terminology used in this text/workbook differs from the standard anatomy-physiology approach because of the emphasis on word building and word element understanding skills required by all medical support personnel. It is not intended to be an anatomy and physiology text because most support staff do not require an intricate knowledge of, for example, the names of each nerve in the hand or the names of every bone in the foot. Rather, the focus is on on-the-job application of medical words through proper pronunciation and spelling for all clerical and support personnel in the field.

Some areas are not covered. Because laboratory equipment and surgical instruments are highly specialized, they are not dealt with in this text. Abbreviations are another topic not addressed in this text because each area of medicine has very specific and specialized abbreviations; moreover, some abbreviations are favored by only some physicians and in some geographical areas. While s with a line over it ($\bar{s}$) is consistently used to mean without, and c with a line over it ($\bar{c}$) means with, AROM indicates either active range of motion or artificial rupture of membranes, depending on the specialty. Students will rapidly acquire the abbreviations used in the area of medicine in which they are working, and all medical dictionaries list the standard abbreviations.

INTRODUCTION

Medical terminology is the tool required for the understanding, transcription, and pronunciation of the majority of not only medical terms, but also words used in everyday conversation and reading. For example, *sub* is always defined as meaning under or below, whether you are referring to a *sub*marine (under or below the ocean) or *sub*costal (of or pertaining to under or below the rib). *Tele* always means far away, or at a distance, whether used in *tele*scope (an instrument to examine something far away or at a distance) or *tele*metry (measurement far away or at a distance). *Mega* means very or exceptionally large—*mega*phone is a sound or voice that is very or exceptionally large, while a *mega*colon is an exceptionally or very large colon.

Basic Medical Terminology Concepts is a complete system of word analysis for the study of terms and/or words related to any type of medically related industry. Medical terminology is used to describe all components of the body in both the normal and abnormal state. It includes diseases and diagnostic methods used in identifying them, as well as their causes and treatments, whether surgical, medical, pharmaceutical, or a combination thereof, and also includes injuries and laboratory techniques, as well as equipment used in the laboratory and in patient rehabilitation. Although the vocabulary is enormous (picked up a comprehensive medical dictionary lately?), the majority of these words use the same bits and pieces covered in and learned from this text. These bits and pieces are called prefixes, suffixes, and roots or stems and are the building blocks of medical

1

terminology. By using the proper combination, in the proper order, one can "create" a word having either a very specific or a very ambiguous meaning, depending on its usage.

Many of the word pieces found in this text are ones already known or familiar. Medical words are "read" in a different way—you define the suffix first, then the prefix, and then the root (anesthesia: *ia* the suffix, meaning condition of, *an* is the prefix, meaning without, and *esthes* is the root, meaning sensation or feeling—thus, anesthesia is a condition of having no sensation or feeling). If there is no suffix, then you start with the prefix (postpartum = *post* means after, *partum* means birth or delivery, or after birth or delivery). If there is no prefix, then read the suffix and then the root (cardiology: *-ology* is the study of; *cardi* means heart). The brand name Magnavox literally means a large (*magna*) voice (*vox*). Other examples include Chloraseptic (named when it came, of course, only in green)—of, pertaining to (*ic*) something green (*chlor*) without (*a*) germs (*sept*). Many more examples are found in the next section, Self-defining Words.

When using terminology, familiarity with the entire word, both alone and in its given context (because some word pieces have more than one literal meaning), is essential. Understanding what the word means ensures accurate transcription, translation, and application. The focus of the text is on learning exact meaning and spelling of word pieces, as well as correct pronunciation of each word (even though the person dictating a word may not always pronounce it correctly). This skill enables anyone to understand and spell words used in dictation, even though the dictator may, at times, combine word elements to describe a specific situation and thereby indulge in "create-a-word." Occasionally, this new word will come into common usage through the publication of manuscripts in a particular field. Knowledge of prefixes, suffixes, and root/stem words enables the typist to understand newly created words and type them correctly.

Word definitions are learned through dexterity in breaking words into easily learned and understood components. As a rule, each word is made up of one or more roots or stems, and the attachment of the describing prefix(s) and/or suffix(es), which add information to the root(s) by adding a full and complete description of the root word itself, stating how, when, where, or why things were done or happened. Analyzing a medical word is similar to diagramming a sentence. The primary reason to learn medical terminology by this system is to enable anyone to see or hear any large medical word and then be able to break it down into familiar, easily defined and understood components. Longer words are actually easier to define because they have more syllables and thus more recognizable word pieces. One can make an educated guess at the meaning of the unknown word pieces or can define the word through using known components and context. Self-defining Words gives everyday word examples of this. Some words will be of few syllables and therefore seem easy to break down. Do not let long words put you off; they are often equally easy to understand, for by deciphering several word parts or sections you already know, you can make an educated guess about the complete definition from context, as well as find the words in a dictionary when you proofread.

Spelling of these words/word elements is of primary importance. The misunderstanding of a pronunciation, the changing of one letter, or the omission of a single letter can change the meaning of a word or even reverse the meaning. A prime example is pt**o**sis (dropping of an organ) and pt**y**sis (spitting or saliva). Changing the *o* to a *y* is a major difference. Another common error occurs with words that sound alike (a homophone—*homo* means same, *phone* means sound or voice). Il**i**um is the lateral (*latero* means side, *al* means of or pertaining to) part of the hip bone, while il**e**um is the distal (pertaining to the furthermost from the point of attachment, or last) portion of the small intestine. Chapter 1, Pronouncing and Spelling Medical Terms, teaches pronunciation and spelling rules for many words. This is possible through the memorization of a few rules. These rules, like most, have exceptions, but learning them will help in both spelling and pronunciation.

Although it is possible to pick up an extensive medical vocabulary after a period of years in a medical environment, it is far easier to learn the lingo by memorizing the bits and pieces (i.e., prefixes, suffixes, and roots or stems) and being able to put them together in the proper sequence or order.

The word elements in Chapter 3, Previewing Prefixes, and Chapter 5, Getting Down to Roots, are listed in their most commonly used divisions. These classifications do not mean that once a word part is pigeonholed as a prefix it will always be found as the first syllable in a word or can never be used as a suffix or root. These divisions merely serve as a method to simplify the learning process. Chapter 4, Suffering Suffixes, uses several root words with a suffix attached, particularly when the suffix is commonly associated with the root as one commonly used word, as in *emia*—a condition of the blood. This attachment to a root also makes it easier to remember what two- or three-letter suffixes mean. Some word pieces are used in just one system, but the majority are used in several systems as a descriptive word piece to describe the function, illness, or problem of multiple systems and their effects on one another.

A variety of exercises are included in each chapter. Some are just for fun, whereas some take a lot of thought. Some (e.g., the crossword puzzles) include words other than medical words, and some (multiple choice questions) may have made-up or misspelled (thus incorrect) "garbage" words.

This is done to make sure not only the definition but the spelling is carefully checked.

Making flash cards, using a different color for prefixes, suffixes, roots or stems, and internal organs, is highly recommended as a study aid. Write the word element on the front and the definition on the back. The more the cards are used, the easier the words become. Once a term is memorized, that card can be removed from the stack, so review is of words the student has trouble remembering. These words are the building blocks, or components, used most often in a majority of frequently used medical words. Some students may want to tape record these word elements, along with their definition, and listen to them while in the car or at home.

On completion of this book, including all exercises, the student will have a working knowledge of most medical words, as well as the skills required to learn new words found in specific work situations. The knowledge that a "five-dollar word" is nothing more than a combination of small bits of words whose meanings are already known should provide a great deal of self-confidence.

There is one primary rule to remember: If in doubt about the spelling of any word, look it up. Don't be afraid to ask questions. That's how smart people get smart—they always ask if they don't know.

PRETEST

Match the best lettered definition with the numbered word.

_____	1.	antero	a.	pus
_____	2.	hetero	b.	under, low
_____	3.	hypo	c.	in front
_____	4.	intra	d.	death
_____	5.	lepto	e.	before
_____	6.	medio	f.	bone
_____	7.	mega	g.	exceptionally large
_____	8.	angio	h.	sleep
_____	9.	narc	i.	between
_____	10.	necro	j.	thin
_____	11.	laparo	k.	from, away
_____	12.	abs	l.	fast
_____	13.	ortho	m.	different
_____	14.	pan	n.	man
_____	15.	pyo	o.	within
_____	16.	semi	p.	vessel
_____	17.	ad	q.	over, high
_____	18.	tachy	r.	freeze, cold
_____	19.	hyper	s.	partly, about half

_____	20.	vari	t. straight
_____	21.	inter	u. middle
_____	22.	brady	v. slow
_____	23.	cryo	w. near, toward
_____	24.	ante	x. all
_____	25.	andro	y. loins, abdomen
_____	26.	osteo	z. different

Fill in the blanks.

27. Adenopathy is a disease of a _____.

28. 29. A lipochilectomy is the _____ of a fat

_____ .

30. A cholecystectomy is the surgical removal of the _____.

31. 32. Hematuria is _____ in the _____.

33. 34. Histology is the _____ of _____.

35. 36. Keratosis is a _____ of the _____.

37. An instrument to examine the abdomen is called a _____.

38. Under the tongue is _____.

39–41. Osteoarthritis is _____ of the _____ and

_____ .

42. The word meaning pertaining to the ear is _____.

Fill in the blanks.

43. 44. Thrombosis is a _____ of the _____.

45. Psychogenic means _____ by the mind.

46. 47. Rhinorrhea is a _____ from the _____.

48. 49. Tinea pedis is _____ of the _____.

50. 51. Afebrile means _____ _____.

Fill in the blanks with the name of the proper medical or surgical specialist.

52.   Surgery on the nervous system _____

53.   Surgery on diseases of the mouth _____

54.   Treatment of the female reproductive system _____

55.   Treatment of the aged _____

56.   Treatment of cancers and malignancies _____

57.   Treatment of a blood disease _____

58.   Treatment of the stomach/intestines _____

59.   Treatment of diseases of the rectum _____

60.   Treatment of infertility in men _____

61.   Counseling for inherited diseases _____

62.   Treatment of hormonal problems _____

Match the best lettered definition with the numbered word.

_____	63.	amphi	a.	tooth
_____	64.	cuti	b.	tongue
_____	65.	cephalo	c.	right
_____	66.	linguo	d.	white
_____	67.	pyelo	e.	difficult, painful
_____	68.	dextro	f.	red
_____	69.	thrombo	g.	cause
_____	70.	erythro	h.	about, both sides
_____	71.	myco	i.	outside, away
_____	72.	cilia	j.	fungus
_____	73.	ora	k.	opening/mouth
_____	74.	etio	l.	clot
_____	75.	alb	m.	fungus
_____	76.	tinea	n.	head
_____	77.	ambi	o.	lip
_____	78.	dys	p.	small hair, eyelash
_____	79.	chilo	q.	blood vessel, vessel, duct
_____	80.	ex	r.	both
_____	81.	dent	s.	renal pelvis
_____	82.	vaso	t.	skin

Multiple choice: Select the best answer(s).

_____ 83. Choledocho means _____ duct or tube.
  (a) bile
  (b) liver
  (c) egg
  (d) all of above
  (e) none of above

_____ 84. Ureto refers to
  (a) joint.
  (b) artery.
  (c) man.
  (d) all of above
  (e) none of above

_____   85.   The word metro also means

    (a)   womb.

    (b)   hystero.

    (c)   uterus.

    (d)   all of above

    (e)   none of above

_____   86.   The large intestine is called

    (a)   laparo.

    (b)   gastro.

    (c)   colo.

    (d)   all of above

    (e)   none of above

_____   87.   Colpo is

    (a)   colon.

    (b)   vagina.

    (c)   rib.

    (d)   all of above

    (e)   none of above

_____   88.   Myo means

    (a)   bone marrow.

    (b)   muscle.

    (c)   spinal cord.

    (d)   all of above

    (e)   none of above

_____   89.   The large pelvic bone is called

    (a)   illeo.

    (b)   ilio.

    (c)   ileo.

    (d)   all of above

    (e)   none of above

_____   90.   Broncho means

    (a)   stomach.

    (b)   mouth.

    (c)   abdomen.

    (d)   all of above

    (e)   none of above

_____ 91.   Orchi means
             (a)   prostate.
             (b)   testicles.
             (c)   ovary.
             (d)   all of above
             (e)   none of above

_____ 92.   The oviduct is also called
             (a)   fallopian tube.
             (b)   salpingo.
             (c)   egg passage/tube.
             (d)   all of above
             (e)   none of above

_____ 93.   The word for intestine is
             (a)   illeo.
             (b)   ilio.
             (c)   entero.
             (d)   all of above
             (e)   none of above

_____ 94.   The word for eye is
             (a)   otic.
             (b)   oto.
             (c)   ophthalmo.
             (d)   all of above
             (e)   none of above

_____ 95.   Myelo means
             (a)   bone marrow.
             (b)   muscle.
             (c)   spinal cord.
             (d)   all of above
             (e)   none of above

_____ 96.   Ano means
             (a)   appendix.
             (b)   man.
             (c)   anus.
             (d)   all of above
             (e)   none of above

_____   97.   The word for nerve is
        (a)   neuro.
        (b)   naso.
        (c)   nevoid.
        (d)   all of above
        (e)   none of above

_____   98.   The word for artery is
        (a)   arterio.
        (b)   arthro.
        (c)   phlebo.
        (d)   all of above
        (e)   none of above

_____   99.   Which of the following refer to the kidney?
        (a)   ren
        (b)   nephro
        (c)   renal
        (d)   all of above
        (e)   none of above

_____   100.   Cranio means
        (a)   encephalo.
        (b)   skull.
        (c)   cephalo.
        (d)   all of above
        (e)   none of above

SELF-DEFINING
WORDS

The following are examples of medical "words" (prefixes, suffixes, and roots or stems) also used in everyday conversation. You know what the word means, but are not sure why, or that there is an association with medical terminology. These words are composed of a combination of prefixes, suffixes, and roots or stems. They are defined by giving first the suffix, then the prefix, and finally, the root. If there is no suffix, then you start at the prefix (or the first part of the word) and keep going.

Word	Elements of Word Example		
taxidermist	taxi(s) = arrangement	derm = skin	ist = one who
telephone	tele = far away		phone = sound or voice
microscope	micro = small		scope = instrument to examine
phonograph	phono = sound, voice		graph = line, drawing, a record
centipede	centi = hundred		ped(e) = foot/feet
transcontinental	trans = across	continent = continent	al = of, pertaining to

Word	Elements of Word Example		
acrobat	acro = top, height		bat = one who walks or haunts
automobile	auto = self		mobile = move
astronaut	astro = star		naut = ship, sailor, sail
stenographer	steno = narrow		graph = lines, drawing, record
cryptographer	crypt(o) = hidden		graph = lines, drawing, record
tachometer	tach(o)(y) = fast		meter = to measure, instrument to measure
diameter	dia = across		meter = to measure, instrument to measure
lunatic	luna = moon		tic = of, belonging to
telemetry	tele = far away		metry = to measure, measurement
periscope	peri = around		scope = instrument to examine
prenatal	pre = before	nat = birth	al = of, pertaining to

PRONOUNCING AND SPELLING
MEDICAL TERMS

1

Medical terms often seem hard to pronounce, particularly when seen in print but never or seldom heard or spoken. Through the study of prefixes, suffixes, and roots or stems, and by the careful pronunciation of each word element, pronunciation will improve daily, and spelling skills will be enhanced. What follows are some rules and shortcuts that will be helpful. When reviewing the examples given, write in words that are in your current vocabulary using the same rules. This will assist you in remembering the rules. One of the most important rules to make pronunciation (and thus spelling) easier is to remember to read vowel to vowel in the word, and always pronounce each and every vowel.

CONSONANTS

Ch Ch has the sound of a hard *k*, as in **chronic** and **pachyderm**, unless the word is not Greek based. *Note*: The language derivatives of all medical words are listed in medical dictionaries.

Ps You only hear and pronounce the *s*, as in **psychiatry** and **psychology**. *Note*: Root words beginning with *psy* refer to the mind.

Pn Only the *n* sound is heard, as in **pneumonia**, unless there is a prefix before the word. In that case, you will hear the *p*, as in **apnea**. *Note*: Root words beginning with *pn* refer to lung, air, breath, or breathing.

C and **G**   These have the soft sounds of *s* and *j*, respectively, before *e, i,* and *y* in words of both Greek and Latin origin, as in **cycle** and **cytoplasm**, and **giant** and **generic**. The most notable exception to this rule is **gynecology**, which has a hard *g*. **C** and **G** have a harsh sound before all other vowels and letters, as in **cast, cardiac**, and **climb**, and **gastric, gonad**, and **grand**.

VOWELS

All vowels are pronounced, with either a long or short sound, going from vowel to vowel to vowel (e.g., pa-tho-gen). Remember what the vowels are—and then include *y* in your list: *a, e, i, o,* and *u*, plus *y*. When a word ends in a vowel , including *y* (unless it is an *a*), it is pronounced with a long sound, as in **rete** (ree-tee). The *a* is short, like *uh*, in words like **amnesia, anoxia, carcinoma, dyspepsia, dysuria, edema,** and **hematuria**.

If there is a vowel in the last syllable of a word, the pronunciation is short, as in **antibiotic**, with the exception of *es*, which is pronounced like *ease*, as in **caries** and **herpes**.

Ae and **oe**   These are normally pronounced as *ee*, as in **orthopaedic** (European spelling of *orthopedic)* and **Aesop**.

Ai   This is pronounced with a short *a*, as in **aide** and **airway**.

Au   **August, aura,** and **automobile** are good examples of the *au* pronunciation.

Eu   This sounds like a hard *u*, as in **euthanasia** and **eustachian** tube.

Ei   You only use a long *i* sound, as in **Einstein**.

E and **Es**   These are commonly used as word endings and are usually pronounced as a separate syllable, as in **rete** (ree-tee) and **herpes** (her-peez). The most notable exception to this is the root word **cele** (a swelling, sac, or hernia) and is pronounced like *seal*.

I   This is used at the end of a word to form a plural (see below) and is pronounced as a separate syllable, with a long *i*, as in **alveoli, cacti, glomeruli**, and **fasciculi**.

Oe   You normally pronounce this as a long *e*, as in **foetal** (European spelling of *fetal*), and find this most often in words used in European literature.

FORMING PLURALS

While everyone is familiar with adding an *s* or *es* for plural endings in most English words, the Greek- and Latin-based words (which are the basis for the majority of medical words, as well as French, Spanish, Italian, and Portuguese) become plural by making these changes to the endings:

ae (oe)   Pronounced with a long *e*. A word ending in a singular may become one ending in *ae* for the plural, as in **fasciae** from **fascia**.

ata   Words ending in *a* (singular) may end in *ata* in the plural form, as in **adenomata** from **adenoma**.

ia   Changing the **cranium** (head) to more than one head (**crania**) is as easy as changing the *ium* to *ia*. *Note*: There is a suffix, *ia*, which means a state, condition or disease, as in **anesthesia**.

I   When the singular form of a word ends in *us*, as in **glomerulus**, it becomes a plural by removing the *us* and adding an **i**—the one most are familiar with is **cactus** to **cacti**.

SPELLING RULES

All of the rules for pronunciation and formation of plurals are necessary for the proper spelling and pronunciation of medical words. Proper pronunciation of the terms will also assist you to spell them more easily and more accurately. However, you must consult a medical dictionary if you are not sure of the spelling. In medical terminology, as in everyday English, there are numerous exceptions to the rules, and a misspelled word can change the entire meaning of a report or diagnosis. Thus, phonetic spelling has no place in medicine. Furthermore, some terms are pronounced alike but spelled differently (homophones, meaning having the same sound). For example, ileum is a part of the small intestine, but the ilium is part of the pelvic bone. Maid/made and deer/dear are two everyday examples of homophones.

Remember—when in doubt, look it up—that's what dictionaries are for.

BODY AND DISEASE
SCIENCES
2

STUDY OF THE BODY

There are six primary branches of medical science that deal with the study of the body:

anatomy
physiology
pathology
embryology
histology
biology

By memorizing the sentence All People Plan Extra Happy Birthdays, you can remember the branches.

Anatomy

This is the study of the structure of the body and the relationship of its parts. In some medical schools, the Department of Anatomy is now the Department of Cellular and Structural Biology. Translated literally, anatomy means to cut (*tomy*) throughout (*ana*); thus, the term is derived from the fact that human body structure is largely learned through dissection.

Physiology

Ology means the study of and *physio* refers to the relationship to nature—thus, physiology is the study of normal functions and activities of the body.

Pathology

Path is a root meaning disease or suffering. When combined with *ology* (the study of), you have the definition of pathology—the study of the changes caused by disease/suffering in the structure or functions of the body. This specialty deals primarily with tissue samples and organs removed either during a surgical procedure or **autopsy** (sometimes called **necropsy**). Through study of that tissue, the disease and pathogens (*gen* means cause or produce) are identified. The results provide the family and physician with a definitive diagnosis and often guide disease management.

Embryology

Embryology is the study of body development from the time the *ovum* (female reproductive cell) unites with the *sperm* (male reproductive cell). This union results in an *embryo*, representing the developing human from one week after conception through the second month, and this specialty covers that time frame. After the end of the second month, the developing human becomes and is referred to as a *fetus*.

Histology

Histo means tissue, and histology is the microscopic study of the minute (small) structure, composition, and function of normal cells and tissues.

Biology

Bio means life, and biology includes the study of all forms of life. This discipline encompasses the study of plant and animal life, including human beings.

BIOLOGICAL STRUCTURE AND FUNCTIONS

All living things (biological structures) are composed of **cells**, which make up **tissues** (groups of cells similar in nature). Tissues make up **organs**, which are groups of tissues working together to perform a specific function. Organs make up **systems**, which are a combination of organs working for a specific purpose. This forms the basic framework for all medical disciplines and specialties.

BASIC SYSTEMS

A **basic system** is a combination of organs working together.

Cardiovascular System—Circulatory System

Cardio is a root word for heart, and *vas* refers to vessels. The heart and blood vessels providing blood transport and nourishment to all body parts comprise this system. This area is treated by specialists in Cardiovascular Disease, such as Cardiologists, Cardiovascular Surgeons, Thoracic Surgeons, and Vascular Surgeons.

Endocrine System

The endocrine system is composed of glands that produce hormones. **Hormones** are secretions that go through the blood stream and act as chemical messengers to all body organs. They send instructions for a variety of things, such as growth, sexual attributes and reproduction, mental status, personality traits, and "flight or fight" instincts. These glands include the thyroid, parathyroid, adrenal, ovaries, testes, etc. Some of these glands are also part of the function of other systems, such as reproduction. Endocrinology and Reproductive Endocrinology are the primary specialties for this system.

Gastrointestinal System—Digestive System

This system covers ingestion (eating), digestion (food absorption or digestion through the stomach, or *gastro*), absorption (through the small and large intestines) of food nutrients, and excretion (elimination of waste material from the intestines through the rectum and anus). Gastroenterologists treat the stomach and intestine, and Proctologists treat the rectum and colon, with some duplication of treatment between them.

Genitourinary System

Genito means genitals (see male reproductive system) and *urin* means urine. This system includes two kidneys (which make urine), two ureters (which transport urine from the kidney to the bladder), the bladder (which stores the urine), and the urethra (which transports urine from the bladder to excretion). In the male, the prostate (which makes a fluid so sperm-containing semen is liquefied) and genitals are part of this system. The prostate gland surrounds the bladder neck and the urethra. See Reproductive System. Urologists and Nephrologists are the primary specialists for this system, although Reproductive Endocrinology occasionally treats male reproductive problems.

Integumentary System—Skin System

This system consists of skin, which covers and protects the body and regulates body temperature, excretion, and sensation. Dermatologists are the primary specialists of this system.

Lymphatic System

Lymph is one of the three main types of body fluid (the others being blood and tissue fluid). Lymph is colorless and odorless and circulates within the lymphatic system. It consists primarily of water (95%) and components of blood plasma as well as lymphocytes (lymph cells). This system takes blood plasma as it seeps through capillary walls to the tissues, where it becomes tissue fluid. It is drained and collected by the lymphatic system, where it becomes lymph, and eventually returns to the blood, where it becomes plasma once again. This system is responsible for the exchange of protein and fluid (with the blood) from body tissue, as well as protecting the body from pathogens (something causing or producing disease). This system is treated by a variety of specialists, including Cytologists, Hematologists, Surgeons, and Oncologists because problems in it can arise from a variety of illnesses.

Muscular System—Musculoskeletal System

Muscles, which provide force for body motion and are attached to the skeletal system, make up this system. As stated above, sometimes the Muscular System is combined with the Skeletal System to form the Musculoskeletal System. This system is treated by either Orthopedics or a subspecialty (like Rheumatology) concerned with particular muscle disorders.

Nervous System and Five Special Senses

All nerves in either the voluntary or involuntary nervous system and the five special senses (touch, taste, smell, seeing, and hearing) interact. They give the body and brain an awareness of the environment and enable the body to react to changes in it. Neurologists and Neurological Surgeons are the primary specialists for the Nervous System. The special senses are treated by specialists in each sense, i.e., Ophthalmology (sight), Otologists or Otorhinolaryngologists (hearing), etc.

Respiratory System

Re means again, and *spire* means breath or breathe. The Respiratory System focuses on breathing and the organs used for breathing, primarily the lungs. The lungs absorb oxygen from the air and provide it to the blood and excrete carbon dioxide, releasing it from the body. A specialist in Pulmonary Disease is the physician treating this system.

Reproductive System

The reproductive system provides the mechanics for fertilization (the union of the *ova* and *sperm*, or germ cells), and the production of sexual hormones through the *gonads* (sex glands—*ovaries* in women, *testes* in men). This system is further broken down into Female and Male Reproductive Systems.

Female reproductive system   This consists of the ovaries, fallopian tubes (oviducts), uterus, cervix, and vagina. They are responsible for production of hormones and provide facilities for reproduction and the production of hormones for lactation (for milk production in the breasts) to nourish the infant. This system is treated by a Gynecologist (*gynec* means woman).

Male reproductive system   The external genitalia (penis, testes, and scrotum), accessory glands (prostate, seminal vesicles), and ducts leading from the prostate to the urethra are the components of the male reproductive system. Because it is involved with the genitourinary system through the urethra, Urologists are the specialists normally treating the male reproductive system. However, in the event of infertility problems, a Reproductive Endocrinologist may become involved in treatment of this system.

Skeletal System—Musculoskeletal System

This system encompasses all bones, the framework of the body. Bones provide support for organs and also furnish places of attachment for muscles. It is occasionally combined with the Muscular System, and called the Musculoskeletal System. It is primarily treated by Orthopedists (literally, ones who straighten feet).

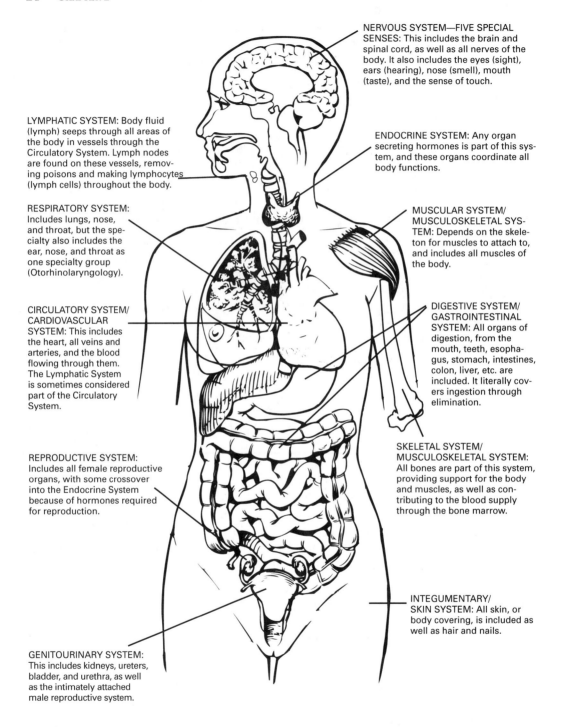

NERVOUS SYSTEM—FIVE SPECIAL SENSES: This includes the brain and spinal cord, as well as all nerves of the body. It also includes the eyes (sight), ears (hearing), nose (smell), mouth (taste), and the sense of touch.

LYMPHATIC SYSTEM: Body fluid (lymph) seeps through all areas of the body in vessels through the Circulatory System. Lymph nodes are found on these vessels, removing poisons and making lymphocytes (lymph cells) throughout the body.

ENDOCRINE SYSTEM: Any organ secreting hormones is part of this system, and these organs coordinate all body functions.

RESPIRATORY SYSTEM: Includes lungs, nose, and throat, but the specialty also includes the ear, nose, and throat as one specialty group (Otorhinolaryngology).

MUSCULAR SYSTEM/ MUSCULOSKELETAL SYSTEM: Depends on the skeleton for muscles to attach to, and includes all muscles of the body.

CIRCULATORY SYSTEM/ CARDIOVASCULAR SYSTEM: This includes the heart, all veins and arteries, and the blood flowing through them. The Lymphatic System is sometimes considered part of the Circulatory System.

DIGESTIVE SYSTEM/ GASTROINTESTINAL SYSTEM: All organs of digestion, from the mouth, teeth, esophagus, stomach, intestines, colon, liver, etc. are included. It literally covers ingestion through elimination.

SKELETAL SYSTEM/ MUSCULOSKELETAL SYSTEM: All bones are part of this system, providing support for the body and muscles, as well as contributing to the blood supply through the bone marrow.

REPRODUCTIVE SYSTEM: Includes all female reproductive organs, with some crossover into the Endocrine System because of hormones required for reproduction.

INTEGUMENTARY/ SKIN SYSTEM: All skin, or body covering, is included as well as hair and nails.

GENITOURINARY SYSTEM: This includes kidneys, ureters, bladder, and urethra, as well as the intimately attached male reproductive system.

MEDICAL AND SURGICAL DISCIPLINES AND SPECIALTIES/SPECIALISTS

Board-certified or **board certification** are terms used to refer to physicians successfully completing specialized programs and testing in their particular field through hospital residencies, which take several years. This extensive training follows their graduation from medical school (receiving their MD [medical doctor] or DO [doctor of osteopathy] degree) and regular internship and/or residency. Board certification is peer recognition that they are well trained and qualified in their field. To maintain certification, physicians are required to keep abreast of new procedures and advances in their field. This is accomplished through continual training via seminars, reading, etc., and, in some instances, periodic testing. Their title is **Fellow** or **Diplomate**, and their Board requires periodic retesting and/or recertification. The majority of the specialties listed have their own Board or College of certification. A board-certified physician usually has a string of initials following MD/DO, such as FACS (Fellow, American College of Surgeons), FACOG (Fellow, American College of Obstetrics and Gynecology), ABO (American Board of Ophthalmology), and FACC (Fellow, American College of Cardiology), signifying which board or college the physician is a fellow or diplomate in. There are even special certifications for speciality procedures.

Medicine and Surgery are the two primary divisions in the practice of medicine, and they each have areas of specialty. Medicine is primarily a diagnostic science and uses a conservative combination of a medical/drug/manipulative approach to disease treatment. Surgery deals with disease process treatment after diagnosis by removal, using surgery, or excision (cutting out). If there is a specialist for an area in Medicine—such as a Cardiologist—there is usually a correlating one in Surgery—Cardiovascular Surgeon. These two areas are further divided into Pediatric (children) specialties because of size of patient, type and size of equipment, and drug reaction variations between children and adults. There are also research specialties in each area, such as Cardiovascular Pharmacology.

Listed below are several specialty areas, with the title of the physician (if appropriate) following.

Aerospace Medicine/Internist

This specialty includes diagnosis and treatment of symptoms and disease caused or affected by gravity/high altitude (*aero*) changes. It also monitors the overall health of astronauts and those involved in the aviation industry. The physician is usually an Internist. Most physicians practicing in this area are in air or space travel facilities, such as NASA or Air Force hospitals or research facilities. See Internal Medicine.

Allergy and Immunology/Allergist—Immunologist

Allergists diagnose, study, and treat abnormal human hypersensitivity to substances that are normally harmless, including pollens, dust, animal hair, plants, and foods or beverages. This field also includes work with diseases produced by allergies, including hay fever, asthma, *urticaria* (hives), eczema, and contact dermatitis. Anaphylactic shock can be caused by a severe allergic reaction. This is produced by any allergen, including foods (e.g., tomatoes and avocados), beverages (e.g., wine, milk), insect bites (e.g., bees, mosquitoes), plants (e.g., poison oak or ivy) and drugs (antibiotics, penicillin). These states involve the immune system. See Immunoallergy and Histology.

Anesthesiology/Anesthesiologist

Anesthesia is the condition of (*ia*) lack of (*an*) feeling or sensation (*esthes*). Artificial or anesthesiologist-induced anesthesia is produced by a number of agents capable of causing partial or complete loss of feeling, sensation, or consciousness. It is either local (restricted to a specific area) or general (the entire body). Anesthetics can be given topically (rubbed on), orally (by mouth), by injection (by needle), or by inhalation (gas). This branch of medicine covers the administration of anesthetics and the condition of the patient from the time anesthesia is given, while under anesthesia, and through awakening. It includes all types of anesthesia; the personnel work in conjunction not only with surgery but most other specialties or practices as well. Obstetrics and Gynecology, Orthopedics, Medicine, and Family Practice are just a few examples.

Bacteriology/Bacteriologist

Bacteriology is the study, usually for diagnostic purposes, of infections caused by an infectious agent (bacteria, germs) in blood and body secretions. The bacteriologist usually works in a research or laboratory environment.

Biochemistry/Biochemist

Biochemists study chemical reactions occurring in living (*bio*) organisms and usually work in a research or diagnostic laboratory.

Biology/Biologist

Biology is the study (*ology*) of life (*bio*), usually at or below the cellular or microscopic level. The biologist usually works in a research or laboratory environment.

Cardiology—Cardiovascular Disease /Cardiologist

Cardio means heart, and *vas* means vessel. These physicians treat all heart-, blood vessel-, and artery-related diseases, using diet, exercise, medicine, or surgery. See Cardiovascular Surgery.

Cardiovascular Surgery/Cardiovascular Surgeon

These surgeons surgically treat some heart-, blood vessel-, and artery-related diseases; they often are involved in transplant surgery. See Cardiology.

Dermatology/Dermatologist

Derma means skin. These physicians deal with the treatment of all skin diseases, including (but not limited to) acne, rashes, melanomas, birthmarks, and moles. The dermatologist also treats skin injuries, such as brown recluse spider bites.

Emergency Room Physician

These physicians have their practice or office in a hospital emergency room, keeping regular office hours and billing patients from there. They treat everything from colds and sore throats to major emergencies such as broken bones, and will call in an appropriate specialist if indicated or requested by the patient; they are not Primary Care Physicians.

Endocrinology/Endocrinologist

Endocrinology is devoted to the study and treatment of the endocrine glands (which secrete hormones) and their effect on patients because of over- or underproduction of these hormones. Diabetes Endocrinology (because of possible effects of diabetes on the entire body) and Reproductive Endocrinology are large treatment areas, and some Endocrinologists specialize in diabetes or fertility problems alone. See Reproductive Endocrinology, Endocrine System.

Epidemiology, Clinical/Clinical Epidemiologist

Epi means on or among; *demi* means people. Epidemiology is the clinical tracing (or following of outbreaks), study, and treatment of factors influencing the frequency and distribution of infections and contagious or recurring diseases in human beings. They include flu epidemics, plague, sexually transmitted diseases (STDs), and acquired immunodeficiency syndrome (AIDS). See Infectious Disease, Public Health.

Family Practice

This is the board-certified area of the old General Practice. The specialty is treatment of the entire family, from newborn through geriatrics. By treating entire families, they have a good general knowledge of the patients' medical and family background and relationships. This is often a key for diagnostics. They are responsible for the day-to-day well being and overall care of their patients and refer them to specialists as indicated; they coordinate patients' ongoing care. These physicians are also known as Primary Care Physicians; with the proliferation of health maintenance organizations (HMOs), they are in the vanguard of patient care. See General Practice, Internal Medicine, Primary Care Physician.

Gastroenterology/Gastroenterologist

This is the study of diseases of the intestine (*entero*) and stomach (*gastro*), and allied treatment, including ulcers and enteritis. Some Gastroenterologists treat the entire gastrointestinal (GI) tract, including the colon (colitis) and rectum (hemorrhoids). See Proctology.

General Practice—General Medicine—Ambulatory Medicine/General Practitioner

These non–board-certified physicians are known as GPs or family doctors and are usually the patient's "regular" or "family" (primary) doctor. They oversee day-to-day care and diagnoses, make referrals to specialists as needed, and keep track of the overall care of the patient. Family Practice is the board-certified form of General Practice. See Internal Medicine, General Practice, Primary Care Physician.

General Surgery/Surgeon

General Surgery is the practice of all types of surgery, with no specific area of specialization. See Surgery.

Genetics/Geneticist

Gen means cause or produce, so *gene* virtually means the cause of and is interpreted as meaning the origin of heredity and the laws governing it. These physicians are found in private practice or research and use family medical histories and laboratory testing to predict possible birth defects or inborn (inherited) diseases. There are two main categories in genetics— clinical and biochemical genetics.

Clinical genetics   This includes counseling of prospective parents for possible inherited (passed down in the family) defects and diseases, such as Huntington's chorea, and chromosomal aberrations causing conditions such as fragile X or Down's syndrome. It also covers immunogenetics, the genetic aspects of antigens and antibodies and reactions that have particular significance in organ transplantation.

Biochemical genetics   This is primarily a laboratory science concerned with the chemical and physical nature of genes and the mechanism(s) by which they control development and maintenance of organisms. Through study, many specific diseases are now known to be inherited. Some examples are sickle cell anemia (hereditary anemia), inborn errors of metabolism (phenylketonuria or PKU), and genetically determined variations of responses to certain drugs like THC, the active ingredient in marijuana, and cocaine.

Geriatrics—Gerontology/Geriatrician

This branch of medicine deals with the care and diseases of the elderly (*geri* means old age). It includes diet and exercise requirements and careful evaluation of medicines for these patients—Internal Medicine or a Family Practitioner for the aging. See Internal Medicine, Family Practice.

Gynecology/Gynecologist

Although sometimes combined with Obstetrics, Gynecology is often practiced alone, which means no obstetrical patients. *Gynec* means woman, and this specialty covers treatment of the female genital tract, including routine Pap smears and mammograms, menstrual irregularities, birth control, and menopause. Gynecologists also often treat their patients for problems of the urinary tract as well. Some subspecialize in Family Planning, Genetic Counseling, and fertility or infertility problems. See Reproductive Endocrinology.

Hematology/Hematologist

Hematology is the science dealing with the study of blood (*hemat*). Hematologists specialize in the diagnosis and treatment of blood diseases, including leukemia and anemias, such as aplastic, iron deficiency, and sickle cell anemia.

Histology/Histologist

In medicine, a Histologist (one who studies tissue) looks into causes of allergies and their effects on tissues. These effects are caused by the release of too many histamines and are treated with antihistamines. Symptoms or diseases covered include allergies, stuffy noses, and bee stings. Some Histologists practice immunoallergy, looking into the causes of allergies and their effects on tissues (like swelling, caused by the release of too many histamines). There are also many other drugs used to treat allergies, including steroids. See Allergy, Immunoallergy.

Hospice Medicine

This growing specialty gives patients (of any age) and their families truthful information about a fatal illness. It provides relief of physical and emotional pain while providing emotional support in the home environment. It allows the patient and the family to make choices and have control over the quality of life. It covers approximately the last 6 months of life, and care is carefully coordinated through the patient's physician (and specialists), hospice physician, nursing services (usually a visiting nurse), psychiatric support, religious support, and pharmacological support.

Immunoallergy/Immunoallergist

Immunology (*immuno* meaning safe, free, or immune) includes the study of body resistance to the effects of a harmful, or noxious, agent, such as pathogenic microorganisms or their poisons, and has several subdivisions. See Allergy, Histology, Immunology.

Immunology/Immunologist

Immunologists are primarily involved in the laboratory aspects of the study and function of the immune system. Organ transplantation actions/reactions, blood banking for transfusing (matching), and, in general, reactions of one body part/fluid to those from another body are all part of this specialty. The specialist makes sure a donated organ matches the immune system make-up of the donee so it won't be rejected. They also ensure donated blood is free from diseases, such as hepatitis or human immuno-deficiency virus (HIV), and is properly labeled as to type and subtypes. See Histology, Immunoallergy.

Industrial Medicine

This specialty is concerned primarily with protection against occupational hazards, such as poisoning by lead or other chemical exposure, and the treatment of those exposures and work-related injuries/accidents. See Family Practice, General Practice, Emergency Room Physician.

Infectious Diseases

This specialty includes study of diseases caused by parasites or virulent organisms. They may be transmitted person to person or insect/animal to person via organism transfer. It covers diseases spread by direct contact with the infectious agent causing it, including body excreta or discharges, indirect contact with objects (drinking glasses, toys, etc.), or other vectors, including rodents, dogs, cats, flies, bats, mosquitoes, ticks, and other creatures capable of transmitting disease. See Epidemiology, Public Health.

Internal Medicine/Internist

This specialty focuses on the diagnosis and treatment of diseases of the internal organs and organ systems of adults. It deals primarily with diagnosis and nonsurgical intervention of diseases and nonsurgical treatment of adults in general by a physician called an Internist. It is not unusual for an Internist to have a subspecialty and practice primarily in that area (e.g., Cardiology). Do not confuse this with the word *intern*, which refers to a graduate medical student receiving medical and surgical training in a hospital before being licensed to practice medicine. These are physicians in training. The term *intern* is gradually being phased out, and the terms *first year resident*, *second year resident*, etc., are replacing it. See Family Practice, Primary Care Physician.

Laryngology/Laryngologist

Laryngo refers to the larynx and Laryngologists treat primarily that area of the throat. See Otorhinolaryngologist.

Maxillofacial Surgery /Surgeon

This surgical field is primarily in the dental field and treats primarily jaws (*maxillo*) and face problems, such as temporomandibular joint syndrome (TMJ). See Oral Surgery.

Microbiology/Microbiologist

This specialty is usually located in a laboratory or research setting and is concerned with diagnosis, treatment, and research of microscopic (very small things seen with an instrument) organisms, including bacteria and molds.

Nephrology/Nephrologist

This specialty treats the kidneys (*nephro*) and is a subspecialty of Urology. Nephrologists are frequently involved in kidney transplant and dialysis procedures and also treat cancer of the kidney. See Urology.

Neurological Surgery/Neurosurgeon

This surgical specialty operates on all aspects of the nervous system (*neuro* means nerve) and works closely with Neurology. Many of these specialists are also Neurologists. See Neurology.

Neurology/Neurologist

Neuro means nerve, and this specialty is the study and treatment of diseases of the nervous system, including all functions and disorders.

Nuclear Medicine/Radiologist, Radiation Oncologist

This branch of Radiology uses radioactive material (radionuclides) in both diagnosis and treatment of a variety of diseases, including thyroid disease and a large variety of cancers. See Radiology.

Obstetrics/Obstetrician

Obstetri literally means midwife, and Obstetricians deliver babies. They take care of the woman from the time of conception through labor, delivery, and the last postnatal checkup, usually 6 weeks after delivery. See Gynecologist, Reproductive Endocrinology.

Occupational Medicine

See Industrial Medicine.

Oncology/Oncologist

Oncos is the Greek word for tumor. Oncologists treat all tumors, not just malignant or cancerous ones.

Ophthalmology/Ophthalmologist

This area covers all diseases of the eye (*ophthalmo*) and associated structures and all treatments of them, including surgery. These physicians also test the eyes and write prescriptions for eyeglasses.

Oral Surgery/Oral Surgeon

This branch of surgery treats problems in the mouth that require surgical attention, including cutting out wisdom teeth. Sometimes, but not always, oral surgeons are also dentists. See Maxillofacial Surgery.

Orthopedic Surgery/Orthopedic Surgeon

Orthopedic Surgery is the surgical treatment of injuries and deformities of the skeletal, and muscular systems. See Orthopedics.

Orthopedics/Orthopedist

Orthopedics literally means straight (*ortho*) feet (*ped*) and is primarily treatment of the skeletal structures (bone) involved in disease processes. These processes include arthritis and trauma (injury) to the bones and connecting joints, muscles, tissues, tendons, etc. See Physical Medicine and Rehabilitation, Sports Medicine.

Otology/Otologist

This specialty treats the ears. See Otorhinolaryngology.

Otorhinolaryngology (ENT)/Otorhinolaryngologist

Oto means ear, *rhino* means nose, and *laryng* means larynx—that's why these physicians and their area is often called ENT, for ear, nose, and throat. They treat all aspects of these organs and sometimes specialize in one or the other. See Otologist, Rhinologist, Laryngologist.

Pain Management

These physicians practice in a clinical setting and often deal with patients referred by another physician for treatment of hard-to-handle pain where standard drug therapies and interventions have failed. They use a variety of treatments for treating pain, including transcutaneous electrical nerve stimulation (TENS) units, biofeedback, hypnosis, distraction techniques, and physical therapy.

Pathology/Pathologist

Pathology is the scientific study of alterations produced by disease (*patho*). These alterations are usually found in a laboratory (where tissue and body fluid samples are sent for diagnostic testing) or research (using specimens from autopsy or cadavers) setting. Pathology subspecialties include:

Clinical   Applied to clinical or patient problem solution

Comparative   Comparing human disease processes with the same process in lower animal species

Experimental   Including study of artificially induced disease processes

Forensic   Legal pathology—the medical "detectives"—a combination of laboratory and research processes to identify anything about or related to the victim or assailant

Oral   Treatment of conditions resulting in or caused by inborn or functional changes in mouth structure

Surgical or tissue and cytological   Study of diseased tissue recovered during examinations (e.g., Pap smears or throat cultures) or surgeries (e.g., tumors, tissue from any operative site). This is the branch of pathology with which most people are familiar.

Pediatrics/Pediatrician

This branch of medicine is devoted to treating and curing diseases of children and is named from *pedi(a)*, for child or education, and *atrics*, for cure. Pediatricians practice well-baby and child care (regular checkups, routine immunizations, etc.), care for newborns, and treat childhood illnesses. Several diseases found in both adults and children are treated in a completely different manner in the very young or very old. Remember the majority of the specialties listed herein also have pediatric specialists in the same fields, as in Pediatric Surgeon, Oncologist, Cardiologist, etc. One rapidly expanding field is Prenatal (before birth) Pediatrics, where diagnosis and treatment are performed on the unborn child or fetus while in utero. **Neonatology** is the science/art of diagnosis and treatment of the newborn infant, or neonate, up to 4 weeks of age.

Pharmacology—Pharmacy/Pharmacologist, Pharmacist

Pharmac means drugs, and this area deals with all aspects of drugs—the laboratory and research setting, clinical setting (office, hospital, and home), and pharmacy. Pharmacology is the theoretical or experimental aspect of drugs and actions/reactions on organisms. This is the primary research arm of drugs; it is often a vital component of new drug development, combined with Clinical Pharmacology.

Clinical pharmacy   This is the area of the professional pharmacist and includes proper preparation and compounding of medicines/drugs, as well as the dispensing of medicines/drugs and medical supplies requiring a physician's prescription.

Clinical pharmacology   This is the bedside (hospital) or home treatment of patients and pertains to (or is founded on) actual observations and treatment of patients. It includes drug dosage adjustments for the patient's particular metabolism, body weight, age, and size, as opposed to theoretical procedures with drugs. It may also involve controlled applications of experimental drugs (trial or field studies) for efficacy (if they work) and side effects (both good and bad). These studies are conducted under rigid criteria in clinical situations.

Physical Medicine and Rehabilitation—Rehabilitative Medicine/Orthopedist, Physical Therapist

Often called PMR, or physiatry, this area uses various methods of physical therapy in disease management. They include thermal (heat) therapy, muscle and nerve stimulation, massage and manipulation of the limbs, working toward the goal of relieving stiffness, minimizing atrophy (*a* means without, *trophy* is nourishment), and promotion of patient mobility. This discipline is also active in making braces and special shoes for specific orthopedic problems. The name is derived from *physic*, meaning physical or natural. This specialty deals with nonsurgical treatment of problems of muscles, nerves, and soft tissue and works closely with Orthopedics. Physical Medicine and Rehabilitation is now called Rehabilitative Medicine in many areas.

Plastic or Reconstructive Surgery/Plastic Surgeon

Plas is a root word for repair, form, or mold. Therefore, a plastic surgeon forms or molds a body part for repair from disease states such as cancer, burn scar reconstruction, eyelid repair for older people with drooping lids, or purely cosmetic reasons.

Primary Care Physician—Internal Medicine—GP—Family Practice

These can be either board-certified Family Practice Physicians, General Practitioners, or Internists. These physicians are usually the patient's "regular" doctor, overseeing day-to-day care and diagnoses, making referrals to specialists as needed, and keeping track of the overall care of the patient. See Internist, Family Practice, and General Practice.

Proctology—Colorectal Surgery/Proctologist—Colorectal Surgeon

This specialty deals with diseases of the rectum (*procto*) (like hemorrhoids), colon (like ulcerative colitis), and related surgeries. It is sometimes a subspecialty of a Gastroenterologist. See Gastroenterology.

Psychiatry—Child and Adolescent/Psychiatrist

See Psychiatry. This deals primarily with children under the age of 18 years.

Psychiatry/Psychiatrist

This branch deals with the diagnosis, treatment, and prevention of mental disorders, and the physician is always an MD. It also covers child psychology, drug and chemical dependence, consultations, and the best known specialty, psychology. There are several subspecialties, including Descriptive Psychiatry (studying and observing external factors that can be seen, heard, or felt) and Dynamic Psychiatry, which studies emotional processes, their origins, and their underlying mental mechanisms.

Psychology/Psychologist

This is the scientific study of mental processes and behavior. It includes abnormal, analytic, clinical, criminal, in-depth and long-term psychoanalysis, experimental, genetic (development of the mind in individuals and with evolution), Gestalt, physiological (facts taught in neurology to show relationships between mental and nerve related), and social aspects of mental life. These physicians are usually a PhD or MD/PhD.

Public Health/Epidemiologist

This field is concerned, primarily, with sanitation and the prevention and control of epidemic diseases, and an investigative tracking of epidemic causes. A prime example is the Centers for Disease Control and Prevention (CDC) in Atlanta, Georgia. Their main focus is on investigations of disease outbreaks, or **pandemics,** throughout the United States, such as drug-resistant tuberculosis (which is reaching epidemic proportions in some cities and areas). Clinical Epidemiologists frequently work in public health and the discipline of infectious diseases is included in this category.

One of the most widely discussed and researched areas today is the study of acquired immunologies (known as induced immunity), which results from antibodies not normally present in the blood. HIV and AIDS are prime examples of abnormal antibodies present; they have no cure although vaccines are looking promising. This field also includes active, cellular, humoral, natural, and passive immunology. See Epidemiology, Infectious Disease.

Pulmonary Disease/Pulmonary Function

This area is concerned with diseases affecting the pulmonary (*pulmo* means lung) system and includes treatment of breathing disorders and lung disease, including (but not limited to) asthma, lung cancers, and emphysema.

Radiology—Diagnostic and Therapeutic (Clinical)/Radiologist

This specialty (*radio* means ray) deals with the use of x-rays, radioactive substances, and other forms of radiation for diagnosis and treatment of diseases. It includes Nuclear Medicine, specialty diagnosis and/or therapy using radioisotopes, etc. This field is also the area of the radiation oncologist, who treats tumors by radiation or radioactive drugs (chemotherapy), and works closely with Oncology. See Nuclear Medicine.

Reproductive Endocrinology—Infertility/Endocrinologist

This specialty is concerned with the functions of both the male (including low sperm counts) and female (including lack of menses and/or egg production and tubal problems) reproductive systems in fertility problems. It works in close association with ongoing research in fertility advancements, including fertility drugs, and laboratory fertilization of retrieved eggs and successful implantation. The area of *in vitro* fertilization (IVF), gamamate intrafallopian tube transfer (GIFT), and zygote intrafallopian tube transfer (ZIFT), as well as the use of surrogates (where the frozen embryo is transferred to the surrogate mother), are part of this specialty. See Endocrinology, Urology, Obstetrics.

Rheumatology/Rheumatologist

Rheumatologists are concerned with chronic diseases marked by pain in joints and/or muscles, or problems commonly called arthritis, rheumatism, osteoarthritis, bursitis, etc.

Rhinology/Rhinologist

Rhino means nose—thus, a Rhinologist is a specialist in all aspects of nose or nasal (*nas* also means nose, *al* means of or pertaining to) disease. See Otorhinolaryngology.

Sociology/Sociologist

Sociology includes the scientific study of human society and of social relationships, organizations, and social change. It also deals with the principles or processes governing social phenomena. Although a social rather than medical science, sociology can relate to the medical field in many ways. One particular area is the coordination of prescribed diets for medical conditions (e.g., diabetes and ulcers) with the cultural and ethnic background of patients, so the diet will be tied into that background.

Sports Medicine/Orthopedist

This specialty treats trauma to bones, muscles, joints, tendons, and tissues caused primarily by *kinesis* (act of movement) or activity; most of the processes treated are sport related. See Orthopedics, Physical Medicine, and Rehabilitation.

Surgery/Surgeon

This discipline treats disease primarily through operative procedures. Specializations are listed throughout by specialty, such as Cardiothoracic Surgery (heart/thorax, chest), General, Oral, Orthopedic, etc.

Thoracic Surgery/Thoracic Surgeon

This specialty is concerned with the surgical treatment of diseases of the chest (*thoraco*) and organs found therein, including the lungs.

Urological Surgery/Urological Surgeon

This is a Urologist specializing in surgery of the urinary tract and the male reproductive tract. See Urology, Genitourinary System.

Urology/Urologist

This specialty covers the entire urinary (*uro* means urine) tract of both men and women, including kidneys, bladder, etc., as well as genital organs and fertility problems in the male reproductive system. See Genitourinary System, Nephrology.

Vascular Surgery/Vascular Surgeon

Vaso means blood vessel, vessel, or duct. This surgeon operates on vessels of the circulatory system.

1. MEDICAL DISCIPLINES FILL IN THE BLANKS EXERCISE

Fill in the blank(s) with the specialty or specialist that most correctly completes the sentence.

1. Heart disease is studied by a/an _____.

2. Chemical reactions occurring in living organisms are studied in ____

    _____.

3. The study of diseases of the intestines and stomach is _____.

4. One of the largest specialties, covering treatment of most disease

    processes, is_____.

5. The area that studies skin disease is _____.

6. Clinical Pharmacology studies the effects of _____ on

    _____.

7. The loss of feeling is _____.

8. Hormonal problems are treated by a/an _____.

9. One treating pregnancy and childbirth is a/an _____.

10. Blood diseases are treated by the specialty of _____.

11. The area of medicine dealing with all aspects of drugs is _____

    _____.

12. Inherited diseases are studied by a/an _____.

13. Infectious diseases are diseases caused by organisms or by a/an ____

    _____.

14. The area of medicine dealing with the removal of any tissue is ____

    _____.

15. The specialty dealing with the overall treatment of children is_____

    _____.

16. Resistance of the body to effects of a harmful agent is treated by

    a/an _____.

17. Hypersensitivity to an agent is studied and treated by a specialist in

    the field of _____.

18. Minute living organisms are studied by a/an _____.

19. Frequency and distribution of infectious, contagious, or recurring

    diseases are studied by a/an _____.

20. Breathing problems are studied by someone specializing in_____

    _____ diseases.

21. The specialty concerned with treatment of the urinary tract is_____

    _____.

22. A graduate medical student completing training in a hospital setting

    is called a/an _____.

23. Rheumatologists work with diseases causing pain in the _____

    _____ or _____.

24. A specialist in women's diseases is a/an _____.

25.   Nuclear medicine is the branch of medicine using radionuclides to

_____ and _____ a variety of

diseases, including thyroid disease and cancers.

26.   The scientific study of alterations produced by diseases is called

_____.

27.   Aging patients are often treated by a specialist in the field of _____

_____.

28.   The branch of medicine using x-rays and diagnosis from them is____

_____.

29.   The scientific study of mental processes and behavior is _____

_____.

30.   One filling a physician's order for a drug is a/an _____.

31.   Specialized treatment at home during the last 6 months of life is____

_____ medicine.

32.   _____ is the specialty for treatment of pain

when standard methods fail.

33.   The specialty responsible for the day-to-day management of patient

care, and for referring the patient to a specialist, is _____.

34.   The specialty treating patients having difficulty getting and/or stay-

ing pregnant is_____.

35.   The specialty using knowledge of kinesis is _____.

2. MEDICAL DISCIPLINES, BRANCHES, TERMS, AND SPECIALTIES EXERCISES

List and define the six branches of science.

1. _____

   _____

2. _____

   _____

3. _____

   _____

4. _____

   _____

5. _____

   _____

6. _____

   _____

Define the following terms and use them in words learned in this chapter.

7. patho _____.

8. bio _____.

9. uro _____.

10. ortho _____.

11. physic _____.

12. ped _____.

13. obstetri _____.

14. histo _____.

15. oto _____.

16. derm _____.

17. gynec _____.

18. ophthalmo _____.

19. psych _____.

20. geri _____.

Name the specialty and specialist treating these organs, problems, or systems. Note: Many of these have more than one possible answer.

1. genitourinary tract _____.

2. heart _____.

3. integumentary system _____.

4. female reproductive tract _____.

5. endocrine system _____.

6. internal organs _____.

7. x-ray interpretation _____.

8. diseases of the mind _____.

9. ears _____.

10. backache _____.

11. male infertility _____.

12. larynx _____.

13. cancer treatment with radionuclides _____.

14. effects of space exploration on astronauts _____.

15. physical therapy in disease treatment _____.

16. male urinary system _____.

17. broken bones _____.

18. problems with the gastrointestinal tract _____.

19. abnormal blood cells _____.

20. heart transplantation _____.

*Name the specialty(ies) treating the following. Note: Open your imagi-
nation—there are several answers for all of these—use them all and
play create-a-word.*

1. deformed foot _____.

2. brain tumor _____.

3. face lift _____.

4. surgical removal of a wisdom tooth _____.

5. sleep prior to surgery _____.

6. wound to the eyeball _____.

7. partial paralysis or muscle atrophy _____.

8.   astronauts at NASA   _____.

9.   injuries incurred at work   _____.

10.   heart attack   _____.

11.   hormonal imbalance   _____.

12.   asthma   _____.

13.   hemorrhoids   _____.

14.   epidemics   _____.

15.   inherited diseases   _____.

16.   nerve disease   _____.

17.   jaw disorders   _____.

18.   chest   _____.

19.   blood vessels   _____.

20.   moles   _____.

3. SPECIALISTS AND THEIR SPECIALTIES PUZZLE

Across

2. Neoplasm specialist
5. Takes pictures of bones
10. Treatment
11. Heart specialist
15. Oxygen ___.
17. Take out (abbr.)
18. Common name for intestines
20. Specialist for women only
26. Urinary tract specialist
29. Mechanical man
30. Item found in atlas
32. Louisiana (abbr.)
33. Cleopatra's "friend"
34. Specialty of disease alterations
36. Leave
37. Lisper's "thing"
41. Hematologist's specialty
42. Overstretch
43. Hormone specialty
45. Taken in midafternoon
46. Otologist's field
47. Physician of Internal Medicine
48. Clue
52. Used in grocery store
53. They care for eyes
57. Long distance (abbr.)
58. It's a ___!
59. Field of students of the mind
61. Ripped
63. Study of life
65. Camping items
66. Neurologist's field
69. Its bite sends you to an allergist
70. Means send/sent
71. Allergists study this
73. What tape does
76. MD organization
77. Proctologist's field
78. Remover of tissue

Down

1. Concern and consideration
2. Neoplasm specialty
3. Flower garland
4. Rhinologist's specialty
5. Balance
6. Who takes care of teeth?
7. Area for a chest surgeon
8. Doctor using operative procedures
9. What some have to a bee sting
12. Something to sweep dust under
13. Nickname for family doctor
14. Those who study life
16. Run in a hurry
19. Pediatrician's patient
21. Shy
22. Obstetrician?
23. Means ear
24. Practitioner of internal medicine
25. Take care of
27. Young boy
28. Fuel for an auto
31. User of a proctoscope ___ and needles
34. Study of body structure
35. Not out
38. Opposite of stop
39. Male fertility doctor
40. Specialty for older people
44. Black
46. Quaker pronoun
48. Impersonal pronoun
49. Study of normal functions
50. Sick
51. Doctor's initials
54. Your male child
55. Drug dispensary
56. Red skin
60. In a hurry
62. Orthopedics area
64. Vigor
67. Estimated time of arrival
68. Desire
72. "___ for the Tummy"
74. I am (contraction)
75.

SPECIALISTS AND THEIR SPECIALTIES PUZZLE

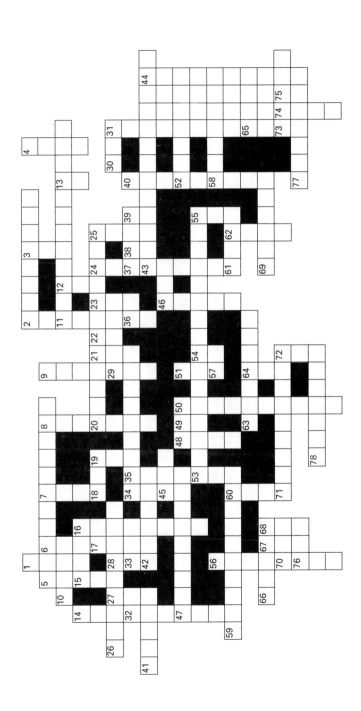

4. BODY AND DISEASE SCIENCES MULTIPLE CHOICE EXERCISES

Select the correct answer(s) and write the letters of your choice in the space provided.

1. All biological structures are composed of
   (a) cells.
   (b) ectoplasm.
   (c) bones.
   (d) blood.

2. Physiology is the study of
   (a) disease.
   (b) body structure and relationship of parts.
   (c) normal functions and activities.
   (d) advanced math.

3. One of the five special senses is
   (a) ESP.
   (b) touch.
   (c) common sense.
   (d) to come in out of the rain.

4. Embryology is the study of
   (a) brain and nerves.
   (b) disease.
   (c) life.
   (d) body development through the 8th week.

5. Histology is the study of
   (a) changes caused by disease.
   (b) tissue structure, composition, and function.
   (c) life.
   (d) events prior to 1960.

6. Biology is the study of
   (a) plants and animals after death.
   (b) all forms of life.
   (c) babies before they are born.
   (d) none of the above.

7. The integumentary system is made up of
   (a) Juicy Fruit.
   (b) papayas.
   (c) gums beneath the teeth.
   (d) none of the above

8. A gynecologist takes care of
   (a) babies.
   (b) old men.
   (c) women.
   (d) teenagers.

9. An anesthesiologist makes you
   (a) have good circulation.
   (b) pass your physical examination.
   (c) feel no pain.
   (d) none of the above

10. Disease processes in aging human beings are studied by
    (a) gerontologists.
    (b) gastroenterologists.
    (c) geneticists.
    (d) gynecologists.

11. The respiratory system includes
    (a) lungs.
    (b) oxygen.
    (c) carbon dioxide.
    (d) the heart.

12. Anatomy is the study of
    (a) life.
    (b) body structure and relationship of parts.
    (c) normal functions and activities of the body.
    (d) disease.

13. The intestines are found in which system?
    (a) female reproductive
    (b) nervous
    (c) gastrointestinal
    (d) skeletal

_____ 14. The skeletal system is made up of
   (a) bones.
   (b) papier-mâché.
   (c) organs.
   (d) all of the above

_____ 15. The urethra is found in which system?
   (a) genitourinary
   (b) integumentary
   (c) cardiovascular
   (d) none of the above

_____ 16. Hormones are produced by which system?
   (a) lymphatic
   (b) integumentary
   (c) skeletal
   (d) endocrine

_____ 17. An allergy is
   (a) hypersensitivity to something.
   (b) hyposensitivity to something.
   (c) influenza.
   (d) atrophy of something.

_____ 18. The fallopian tubes are found in which system?
   (a) female reproductive
   (b) genitourinary
   (c) cardiovascular
   (d) muscular

_____ 19. Infectious diseases are caused by
   (a) bacteria.
   (b) pathogens.
   (c) infectious agents.
   (d) all of the above

_____ 20. Heart disease is treated by a(n)
   (a) endocrinologist.
   (b) hematologist.
   (c) histologist.
   (d) cardiologist.

_____   21.   Pathology is the study of
    (a)   disease.
    (b)   normal cells and tissues.
    (c)   life.
    (d)   body development.

_____   22.   Children are taken care of by
    (a)   gerontologists.
    (b)   podiatrists.
    (c)   pediatricians.
    (d)   pathologists.

_____   23.   Endocrinology is the study of
    (a)   the inside of the brain.
    (b)   bones.
    (c)   vessels and their fluids.
    (d)   glands and hormone secretions.

_____   24.   Hematology is the study of
    (a)   serum.
    (b)   blood.
    (c)   urine.
    (d)   spinal fluid.

_____   25.   Genetics means
    (a)   Levis.
    (b)   blind spots in the eye.
    (c)   the cause or producing.
    (d)   origin of heredity.

_____   26.   The cardiovascular system provides
    (a)   electrocardiograms.
    (b)   romance novels.
    (c)   pacemakers.
    (d)   blood transport and nourishment.

_____   27.   For a broken bone, you would see a
    (a)   plastic surgeon.
    (b)   orthopedist.
    (c)   anesthesiologist.
    (d)   podiatrist.

_____   28.   X-rays are interpreted by
    (a)   rhinologists.
    (b)   anesthesiologists.
    (c)   radiologists.
    (d)   psychiatrists.

_____   29.   A GP is a
    (a)   good person.
    (b)   general pediatrician.
    (c)   general practitioner.
    (d)   general pathologist.

_____   30.   Psychiatry works with disorders of the
    (a)   mind.
    (b)   body.
    (c)   soul.
    (d)   brain.

PREVIEWING
PREFIXES

3

A prefix, by definition, is one or more letters or syllables (you can have more than one prefix in a word) placed at the beginning (*pre* means before, *fix* means to fix) of a word to modify, change, or enhance the root or stem word. After pronouncing the prefix and definition/meaning, draw a slash between the prefix and remainder of the word example(s) so you can visualize each word as being composed of several small pieces. For example, tachycardia becomes tachy/card/ia, a condition of (*ia*) (suffix) a fast (*tachy*) (prefix) heart (*card*) (root). *Note:* Some of the words are roots or stems and are used before another root in the word example.

PREFIXES WITH MEANING AND WORD EXAMPLE(S)

LOCATIONS AND POSITIONS*

Prefix	Meaning	Word Example(s)
acro	top, extremity, height	acrophobia, acrobat
ad	near to, near, toward	adrenal, adverb
ambi	both	ambidextrous
amphi	on both sides, both, about	amphitheater, amphibious
ante	before	antemortem, antepyretic
antero	in front (from *ante*, before), the front	anterolateral

LOCATIONS AND POSITIONS*

Prefix	Meaning	Word Example(s)
crypt	hidden	cryptorchidism, cryptograph, cryptic
dextro	right	ambidextrous, dextromanual
dia	across, through, between, completely	diameter
ec, ecto	on the outside, external	ectoderm, ectogenous
endo	inner, inside, within, inward	endocarditis
epi	upon, among	epidemic, epidermal
eso	within, inward	esophagus, esogastritis
ex(o)	outside, out, away	excise, exocolitis
extra	outside of	extracellular, extrauterine
hemi	half, usually lateral (one side)	hemianalgesia, hemidystrophy
infra	below, beneath	infracostal, infrascapular
inter	between	intercostal, interstate
intra	within	intravenous
ipsi	same, self	ipsilateral
latero	to the side of	lateroversion
levo	left	levorotation, levoversion
medio	middle	mediocre, mediotarsal
meso	middle	mesoderm
opisth(o)	backward, behind, located behind	opisthotic
ortho	straight	orthodontist, orthopnea
para	beside, near, beyond, apart from	paramedian, paralegal, paramedic
peri	around	perimeter, periscope, periotic
post	after	postpartum, postoperative
postero	behind, the back of	posterolateral, posteroanterior
pre	before	prenatal, preventive, premenopausal
retro	behind, located behind	retrolateral, retrolingual
sub	under	subcutaneous, subnormal
super	above, over	superego
supra	over, above	supralumbar

LOCATIONS AND POSITIONS*

Prefix	Meaning	Word Example(s)
tele	far away, distance, at a distance	telemetry
trans	across, through, beyond	transcervical, transfer, transverse, transdermal
vari	different	various

*Several of these terms are commonly used as roots or stems.

TIME

Prefix	Meaning	Word Example(s)
ante	before	antenatal
neo	new	neonatal
post	after	postmortem, postoperative
pre	before	precancerous

NEGATION

Prefix	Meaning	Word Example(s)
a	without, from, away	afebrile
ab	from, away	abduct
abs	from, away	abscise
an	without	anesthesia
anti	against	antipyretic, antidote
de	from, remove	dehydrate, decapitate

NUMBERS, AMOUNTS, AND COMPARISON

Prefix	Meaning	Word Example(s)
ambi	both	ambidextrous
bi	two, double, both	bicuspid, bilateral
brady	slow	bradycardia
di	two, double, both	dicephalous, diphonia
dipl(o)	two, double	diplopia, diplomat

NUMBERS, AMOUNTS, AND COMPARISON

Prefix	Meaning	Word Example(s)
du(o)	two, double	dual, duodenostomy
eu	good, well, normal	euthyroid, euphoria
hemi	half (usually lateral)	hemiplegia, hemisphere
hetero	different	heterosexual
hex(a)	six	hexapod
hyper	over, too much, high	hypertension, hyperventilate
hypo	under, low, too little	hypodermic, hypoglycemia
mono	one, single	mononeural
multi	many	multicellular
pan	all	pandemic, panacea
poly	many, much, excessive amount	polyuria
quadr	four, ¼ th	quadruped, quadrant, quadrantanopia
semi	partly, about or almost half	semiconscious, semicircle
sex(i)	six	sextuplets
tach(o)(y)	fast	tachometer, tachycardia
tetra	four	tetralogy, tetraplegia
tri	three, triple	triangle
uni	one, single	uniform
vari	different	variometer

COLORS*

Prefix	Meaning	Word Example(s)
alb	white	albino
brun	brown	brunette
chloro	green	chlorophyll
chrom(a,o)	color	chromogenic, monochrome
cirrho	orange	cirrhosis
cyano	blue	cyanosis

COLORS*

Prefix	Meaning	Word Example(s)
erythro	red	erythrocyte, erythroderma
leuco	white	leucocyte
leuko	white	leukemia
lute	yellow (refers to corpus luteum, similar to egg yolk)	luteal
melan	black	melanoma
purpur	purple	purpura
xantho	yellow	xanthoma, xanthophyll

*These are root words being used in this chapter at the start of each word as they are descriptive of root words.

SIZE

Prefix	Meaning	Word Example(s)
dolicho	long	dolichofacial
lepto	thin	leptodermic
lipo	fat	liposuction, lipoma
macro	excessively large or long	macronychia
mega	exceptionally large	megacolon
micro	small	microscope

MISCELLANEOUS*

Prefix	Meaning	Word Example(s)
aero	air, gas	aerodontalgia
andro	man	android
auto	self	autolysis, automobile, autobiographical
bio	life	biology, biochemical
dys	difficult, painful	dysfunctional, dysmenorrhea
etio	cause	etiology
eu	good, well, normal	euthyroid, euphoria, euthanasia
febr	fever, fire	febrile, afebrile
gluc(o)	sweet, sugar	glucogenic
glyc(o)	sweet, sugar	hypoglycemia

MISCELLANEOUS*

Prefix	Meaning	Word Example(s)
gyn(o)	woman	gynandrism
gyne(c, co)	woman	gynecology, gynecopathy
hydro	water, water-like fluid	hydroma, hydrocele
lipo	fat	liposuction, lipoderm
mal	bad	malnutrition, malocclusion
narc	sleep	narcotic, narcolepsy
necro	death	necrophobia, necrosis, necrotic tissue
neo	new	neonatal
noct	night	nocturia, noctambulism
nox(i)	injurious agent, act, influence	noxious
nox	night (rarely)	Noxema
path	disease, suffering	pathogen, pathology
pyo	pus	pyorrhea
pyro	fever, fire	pyrogen, pyromaniac
sui	self	suicide

*Several of these terms are commonly used as roots or stems.

POSITIONS AND LOCATIONS

Position	Meaning
anterior	of or pertaining to front of body (*antero* means front)
caudal	of or pertaining to (*al*) the lower portion of the spinal column
cavity	any hollow space
cephalad	toward, near, near to (*ad*) the head (*cephal*)
cranial	of or pertaining (*al*) to the skull (*cranio*)
distal	of or pertaining to (*al*) the furthermost from point of attachment (*dis*)
dorsal	of or pertaining to (*al*) the back of the body or any body part
external	of or pertaining to (*al*) the outside (*ex*)
inferior	below
internal	of or pertaining to (*al*) the inside
lateral	of or pertaining to (*al*) the side (*latero*) of the body or any body part

POSITIONS AND LOCATIONS

Position	Meaning
medial	of or pertaining to (*al*) toward the midline, or middle of body or any body part
midline	imaginary line dividing body/body part into right and left sides through center
parietal	of or pertaining to (*al*) the wall of a body structure
peripheral	of or pertaining to (*al*) near the surface
posterior	the back of the body or any body part (*postero* means back)
prone	lying face down—opposite of supine
proximal	of or pertaining to (*al*) the nearest point of attachment
superior	above, over
supine	lying on back—opposite of prone
ventral	of or pertaining to (*al*) the front of the body or body part
visceral	of or pertaining to (*al*) structures found inside the body

ABDOMINAL DIVISIONS AND REGIONS

The abdomen is divided into four parts, or quarters, called **regions** or **quadrants** (meaning ¼ th). They are shown on the diagram as cross-hatched lines and are called:

    right upper quadrant   left upper quadrant
    right lower quadrant   left lower quadrant

The right or left side of the patient is always the one referred to, not the right or left of the examiner.

The abdominal regions are shown on the diagram as dark dotted lines, with the areas numbered and corresponding to their names and locations as follows:

1. left hypochondriac (front)
2. epigastric (front)
3. right hypochondriac (front)
4. left lumbar (back)
5. umbilical (front)
6. right lumbar (back)
7. left inguinal or left iliac (front)
8. hypogastric or suprapubic (front)
9. right inguinal or right iliac (front)
10. femoral (front)

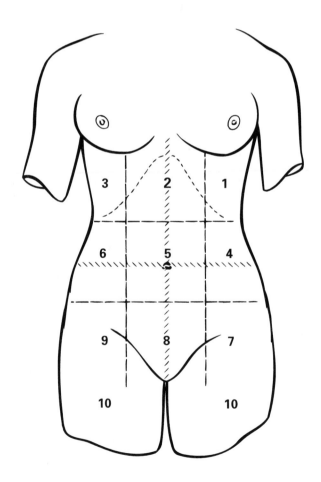

BASIC SURGICAL INCISIONS

This list of incisions includes those most commonly used in abdominal surgeries that are not done laparoscopically. The numbers on the drawing correspond with their names, with a line indicating each incision area. However, all can be anywhere in the region described, with exceptions as indicated.

1. subcostal—of or pertaining to (*al*) under (*sub*) the rib (*cost*). This can be anywhere below the ribs on either side.
2. midline—anywhere up or down the imaginary line showing the exact middle of the body
3. mid-rectus—anywhere in the middle of the rectus muscle
4. upper right rectus—anywhere in the upper right portion of the rectus muscle

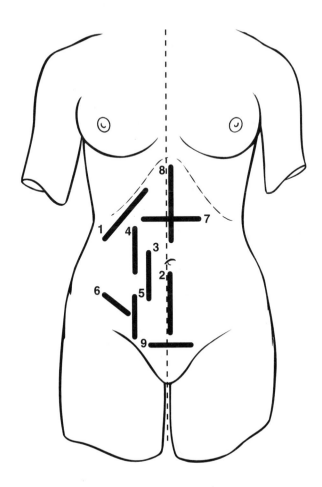

5. lower right rectus—anywhere in the lower right portion of the rectus muscle
6. McBurney's—standard appendectomy site, about 2 inches toward the umbilicus (belly button) from the top of the pelvic bone (ilium)
7. transverse—any incision on the abdomen turning across the abdomen
8. paramedian—any incision near to or toward the median, or imaginary line exactly in the middle of the abdomen
9. suprapubic—anywhere above (*supra*) the pubic bone

POSITIONS FOR SURGERY AND EXAMINATION

The more common positions for surgery and/or examination are listed below.

Dorsal or supine   Lying on back, legs straight, head in line with body, arms alongside body, palms down.

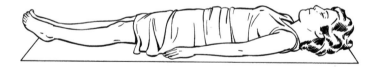

Dorsal recumbent   Lying on back, head in line with body, knees bent at approximately 45°, arms alongside body, palms down.

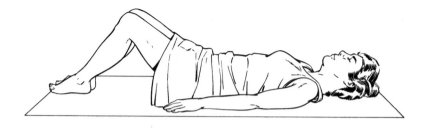

Trendelenberg   Lying on back, knees bent over lower break of table, arms alongside body, palms down, with head and legs flexed lower than middle of body or legs and feet elevated, body supine (as shown in drawing).

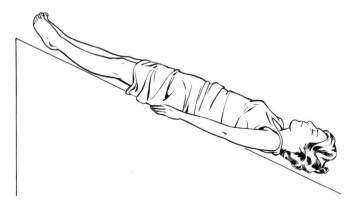

Dorsal lithotomy   On back, arms crossed over chest, knees raised well over buttocks, with feet in stirrups, flexed and rotated outward.

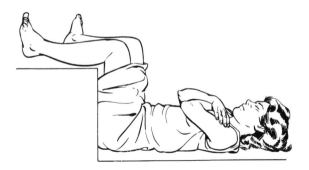

Knee-chest   Chest and side of face down on table, buttocks elevated, knees completely flexed with top of feet on table.

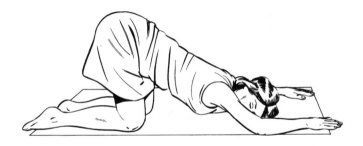

Fowler   Head up, knees flexed 45°, feet down.

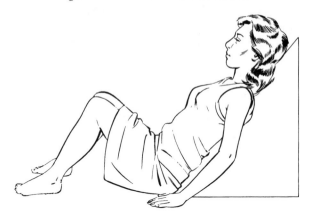

Prone   Face down, opposite of dorsal or supine.

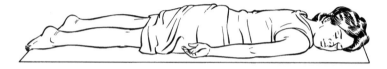

Sims   Lying on left side, knees flexed toward abdomen.

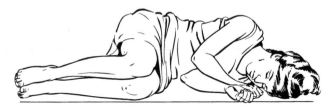

Lateral   Lying on either side, with body at table edge, lower leg slightly flexed, upper leg straight (if a pillow is placed between legs) or fully flexed (as shown) for comfort and ease of examination, with arms outstretched at right angles for support.

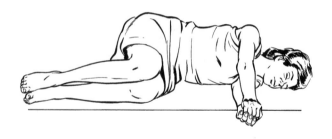

1. POSITIONS AND LOCATIONS MATCHING EXERCISE

Match the following positions and locations in the left column with the definition in the right column.

_____   1. dorsal   a. lying on face

_____   2. supine   b. pertaining to back of body

_____   3. anterior   c. pertaining to front of body

_____   4. peripheral   d. pertaining to the inside

_____   5. distal   e. toward the head

_____   6. external   f. pertaining to head or skull

_____   7. medial   g. pertaining to back of body

_____   8. posterior   h. above

_____   9. cavity   i. pertaining to nearest point of attachment

_____   10. cranial   j. pertaining to near the surface

_____   11. superior   k. lying on back

_____   12. lateral   l. pertaining to farthest from point of attachment

_____   13. prone   m. pertaining to structures found inside body

_____   14. ventral   n. pertaining to front of body

_____   15. visceral   o. pertaining to lower part of spinal column

_____   16. inferior   p. pertaining to toward the midline

_____ 17. cephalad   q. below

_____ 18. caudal   r. pertaining to structure wall

_____ 19. proximal   s. any hollow space

_____ 20. internal   t. pertaining to outside

_____ 21. parietal   u. pertaining to side of body

2. PREFIX DEFINITION EXERCISE

Underline the prefix in each word and define it in the space provided.

1. intravenous _____.

2. retrosternal _____.

3. periotic _____.

4. ectoderm _____.

5. excise _____.

6. supralumbar _____.

7. antenatal _____.

8. prenatal _____.

9. postmortem _____.

10. neoplasm _____.

11. abnormal _____.

12. anesthesia _____.

13. dehydrate _____.

14. hemiplegia _____.

15. hypotension _____.

16. hypertension _____.

17. triangle _____.

18. bradycardia _____.

19. multicellular _____.

20. semiconscious _____.

21. tachycardia _____.

22. bicuspid _____.

23. polyuria _____.

24. leucocyte _____.

25. cyanosis _____.

26. albumin _____.

27. erythrocyte _____.

28. ambidextrous _____.

29. anterolateral _____.

30. posteromedial _____.

31. dextromanual _____.

32. levotorsion _____.

33. lateroversion _____.

34.   mediotarsal_____.

35.   hydrocephalus_____.

36.   malnutrition _____.

37.   biology _____.

38.   etiology_____.

39.   narcotic _____.

40.   micrometer _____.

41.   megacolon_____.

42.   panacea _____.

43.   pyogenic_____.

44.   febrile _____.

45.   aeroplane_____.

46.   dysuria_____.

47.   noctambulism _____.

Define the following.

48.   cavity _____.

49.   proximal _____.

50.   medial _____.

3. MORE PREFIXES DEFINITION EXERCISE

Underline the prefix and define it.

1.   leukemia _____.

2.   perimeter _____.

3.   precancerous_____.

4.   postoperative_____.

5.   abstract _____.

6.   esogastritis_____.

7.   antipyretic _____.

8.   hemianalgesia _____.

9.   intercostal _____.

10.   diphonia _____.

11.   hexapod_____.

12.   brunette _____.

13.   mononeural _____.

14.   anterolateral_____.

15.   opisthotic_____.

16.   diplopia _____.

17.   retrolingual _____.

18.   quadrant_____.

19.   chlorophyll_____.

20. cirrhosis_____.

21. android_____.

22. uniform_____.

23. ambidextrous_____.

24. adrenal_____.

25. transcervical_____.

26. posterolateral_____.

27. superego_____.

28. levorotation_____.

29. mesoderm_____.

30. melanoma_____.

31. purpura_____.

32. diameter_____.

33. necrosis_____.

34. sextuplets_____.

35. pyorrhea_____.

36. euthyroid_____.

37. afebrile_____.

38. neonatal_____.

39. autolysis_____.

40. amphitheater_____.

Define the following terms.

41. posterior _____.

42. inferior _____.

43. visceral _____.

44. peripheral _____.

45. prone _____.

46. external _____.

47. internal _____.

48. parietal _____.

49. caudal _____.

50. cranial _____.

4. PREFIX COMPLETION EXERCISE

Fill in the blanks with the correct prefix.

1. An abnormal fear or dread of height is _____ phobia.

2. *Dual* literally means of or pertaining to _____.

3. The removal by suction of fat is _____ suction.

4. Water of the brain is called _____ encephalosis.

5. The condition of sugar being caused or produced is _____ genic.

6. A condition of the blood with low sugar is hypo _____ emia.

7.   Walking at night (usually in your sleep) is _____ambulism.

8.   Something causing or producing pus is _____genic.

9.   Something removing fever is an _____pyrogen.

10.   A condition of difficult or painful urination is _____uria.

11.   _____dermal means below or under the skin.

12.   A normal, good, or well thyroid is described as _____thyroid.

13.   Behind the tongue is _____lingual.

14.   Heterosexual is of or pertaining to _____sex.

15.   The study of four is _____ology.

16.   Below the scapula is _____scapular.

17.   Across the skin is _____dermal.

18.   A condition of a slow heart is _____cardia.

19.   Of a long face is _____facial.

20.   Of many cells is _____cellular.

21.   Excessively large or long fingernails is _____onychia.

22.   The study of women is _____ology.

23.   One with a madness or compulsion for fires is a _____maniac.

24.   One who uses both hands like the right hand is ambi_____.

25.   A yellow-colored tumor is a _____oma.

26.   A condition of thin skin is _____dermia.

27.   A condition of a fast heart is _____cardia.

28. The killing of self is _____cide.

29. Of many cells is _____cellular.

30. A white cell is called a/an _____cyte.

31. Behind the ear is _____otic.

32. *Periotic* means _____the ear.

33. Something with four feet is called a _____ped or pod.

34. One abnormally afraid of death is _____phobic.

35. One causing a person to have straight teeth is an _____dontist.

36. The condition of having a hidden or undescended testicle is ____

     _____ orchidism.

37. A cure-all is a _____acea.

38. Outside of the cell is _____cellular.

39. Of or pertaining to the same side is _____.

40. To measure from far away or from a distance is _____ metry.

5. PREFIX PUZZLE

ACROSS

2. Difficult, painful
4. White
8. Slow
9. Against
11. Too little, under, low
15. Middle
17. Many, much
19. Red
22. Before
24. Dead
26. He, she, or _____.
27. Upon
28. Behind
29. Cause
30. Water
31. Behind, backward
33. Thin
35. _____ off a branch
36. In front
38. Inner, inside
39. Four
40. Pus
43. White
45. Within
48. Harmful or bad influence
49. Donkey
51. Put it _____
52. Large
54. Above
55. Fever
57. Both

DOWN

1. Half
3. Under
5. Blue
6. Fast
7. Sweet, sugar
10. New
12. Straight
13. Woman
14. Around
16. On the outside
17. After
18. Sleep
20. Behind
21. Too much, over, high
23. Right
24. Night
25. Hidden
30. Nickname for "honey"
32. Four
34. Fever, fire
35. To the side of
37. Bad
40. All
41. Owns
42. Between
44. Left
46. Before
47. Small
49. From, away
50. Above
52. Very large
53. Away
56. Life
58. In the middle

PREFIX PUZZLE

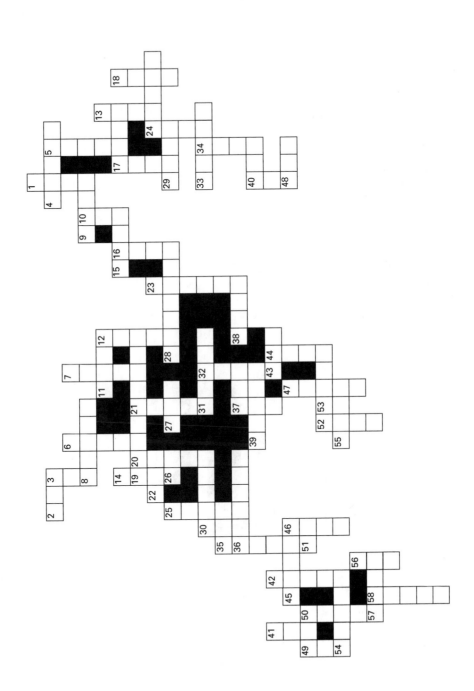

6. ABDOMINAL REGIONS AND INCISIONS PUZZLE

ACROSS

2. Across and above belly button
4. Middle
7. Upper right or left under ribs or cartilage
8. Lower back
9. Up and down near midline
11. Bottom right or left
12. To right of belly button, middle and lower quadrant
13. Above pubic bone
14. Appendectomy incision

DOWN

1. Right or left upper thigh
3. Angle across right to middle upper quadrant
5. Middle upper quadrant
6. Right or left lower quadrant
7. Middle lower quadrant
10. Over pubic bone

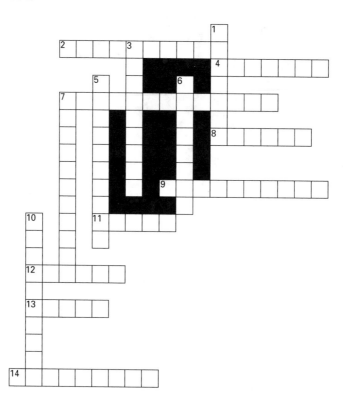

7. PREFIX MULTIPLE CHOICE EXERCISE

Select the correct answer(s) and write the letter(s) of your choice in the space.

_____ 1. A prefix is always found at the
    (a)   end of each word.
    (b)   middle of each word.
    (c)   beginning of each word.
    (d)   the beginning or end of each word.

_____ 2. Super means
    (a)   great.
    (b)   above.
    (c)   below.
    (d)   between.

_____ 3. Semi means
    (a)   about half.
    (b)   at least half.
    (c)   over half.
    (d)   how you cook a steak.

_____ 4. The word(s) for within or inside is/are
    (a)   erythro.
    (b)   endo.
    (c)   external.
    (d)   none of the above

_____ 5. The word(s) for outside is/are
    (a)   extra.
    (b)   poly.
    (c)   ecto.
    (d)   antero.

_____ 6. Dextro means
    (a)   sugar.
    (b)   left.
    (c)   right.
    (d)   both.

_____   7.   Ad means
     (a)   something selling merchandise.
     (b)   white.
     (c)   height.
     (d)   near, toward.

_____   8.   The word(s) for above is/are
     (a)   para.
     (b)   sub.
     (c)   supra.
     (d)   super.

_____   9.   Melan means
     (a)   watermelon.
     (b)   orange.
     (c)   black.
     (d)   green.

_____   10.   The word(s) for upon is/are
     (a)   epi.
     (b)   erythro.
     (c)   lipo.
     (d)   prone.

_____   11.   Sub means
     (a)   across.
     (b)   under.
     (c)   behind.
     (d)   thin.

_____   12.   Necro means
     (a)   black.
     (b)   without.
     (c)   different.
     (d)   dead.

_____   13.   Andro means
     (a)   man.
     (b)   woman.
     (c)   human.
     (d)   child.

_____   14. The word(s) for air is/are
                  (a)   acro.
                  (b)   aero.
                  (c)   ambi.
                  (d)   alb.

_____   15. Dys means
                  (a)   two, double.
                  (b)   brown.
                  (c)   difficult or painful.
                  (d)   simple.

_____   16. Latero means
                  (a)   on the left side.
                  (b)   to the side of.
                  (c)   at the bottom of.
                  (d)   ladder rungs.

_____   17. Etio means
                  (a)   cause.
                  (b)   fever.
                  (c)   around.
                  (d)   outside of.

_____   18. Mono means
                  (a)   kissing disease.
                  (b)   many.
                  (c)   one, single.
                  (d)   more than two.

_____   19. Para means
                  (a)   above.
                  (b)   beside, near, beyond, apart from.
                  (c)   around.
                  (d)   after.

_____   20. Which word(s) mean(s) white?
                  (a)   alb
                  (b)   chro
                  (c)   aero
                  (d)   ad

_____ 21. Hypo means
   (a)   above.
   (b)   beside.
   (c)   low.
   (d)   half.

_____ 22. Neo means
   (a)   old.
   (b)   three.
   (c)   after.
   (d)   new.

_____ 23. Uni means
   (a)   items.
   (b)   one.
   (c)   too much.
   (d)   many.

_____ 24. Antero means
   (a)   in front.
   (b)   to the side.
   (c)   behind.
   (d)   across.

_____ 25. The word(s) for life is/are
   (a)   necro.
   (b)   bio.
   (c)   neo.
   (d)   auto.

_____ 26. Multi means
   (a)   too much.
   (b)   fast.
   (c)   four.
   (d)   many.

_____ 27. Anti means
   (a)   for.
   (b)   against.
   (c)   four.
   (d)   before.

_____   28.   Ex means
(a)   cause.
(b)   upon.
(c)   past.
(d)   outside, away.

_____   29.   Meso means
(a)   middle.
(b)   top.
(c)   bottom.
(d)   none of the above.

_____   30.   Ab means
(a)   white.
(b)   near to, toward.
(c)   from, away.
(d)   large.

_____   31.   The word(s) for two or double is/are
(a)   bio.
(b)   bi.
(c)   tri.
(d)   multi.

_____   32.   An means
(a)   near to, toward.
(b)   before.
(c)   from, away.
(d)   without.

_____   33.   Tetra means
(a)   snake.
(b)   four.
(c)   three.
(d)   many.

_____   34.   Pyo means
(a)   pus.
(b)   fever.
(c)   around.
(d)   much.

_____ 35. Retro means
    (a) before.
    (b) thin.
    (c) behind.
    (d) small.

_____ 36. Tachy means
    (a) improperly dressed.
    (b) fast.
    (c) slow.
    (d) normal speed.

_____ 37. Peri means
    (a) beside.
    (b) around.
    (c) many, much.
    (d) behind.

_____ 38. Ambi means
    (a) against.
    (b) white.
    (c) about, both sides.
    (d) both.

_____ 39. Micro means
    (a) large.
    (b) very large.
    (c) thin.
    (d) small.

_____ 40. Di means
    (a) double.
    (b) triple.
    (c) many, much.
    (d) slow.

_____ 41. Cyano means
    (a) nose.
    (b) blue.
    (c) black.
    (d) yellow.

_____   42.   Opistho means
       (a)   eye.
       (b)   backward.
       (c)   across.
       (d)   straight.

_____   43.   Medio means
       (a)   middle.
       (b)   bad.
       (c)   black.
       (d)   behind.

_____   44.   Abs means
       (a)   near to, toward.
       (b)   white.
       (c)   from, away.
       (d)   before.

_____   45.   Lute means
       (a)   an instrument to examine.
       (b)   white.
       (c)   green.
       (d)   yellow.

_____   46.   Tele means
       (a)   call.
       (b)   far away.
       (c)   describe.
       (d)   across.

_____   47.   Chro means
       (a)   bird.
       (b)   frozen.
       (c)   color.
       (d)   blue.

_____   48.   Inter means
       (a)   between.
       (b)   one.
       (c)   inside.
       (d)   mix.

_____ 49.   Quad means
    (a)   three.
    (b)   four.
    (c)   six.
    (d)   shoe width.

_____ 50.   The word(s) for behind, or located behind is/are
    (a)   retro.
    (b)   meso.
    (c)   endo.
    (d)   supra.

_____ 51.   Hemi means
    (a)   blood.
    (b)   double.
    (c)   half.
    (d)   too much.

_____ 52.   Poly means
    (a)   parrot.
    (b)   many, much.
    (c)   about half.
    (d)   slow.

_____ 53.   Lepto means
    (a)   left.
    (b)   fat.
    (c)   large.
    (d)   thin.

_____ 54.   Ortho means
    (a)   straight.
    (b)   teeth.
    (c)   bone.
    (d)   behind.

_____ 55.   Pan means
    (a)   all.
    (b)   bread.
    (c)   sides.
    (d)   view.

_____   56. Hetero means
            (a)   uterus.
            (b)   too much.
            (c)   same.
            (d)   different.

_____   57. Noct means
            (a)   middle.
            (b)   night.
            (c)   rap.
            (d)   sleep.

_____   58. Febr means
            (a)   pus.
            (b)   woman.
            (c)   fever.
            (d)   sweet.

_____   59. Hyper means
            (a)   not enough.
            (b)   slow.
            (c)   too much.
            (d)   fast.

_____   60. Brady means
            (a)   slow.
            (b)   fast.
            (c)   under.
            (d)   across.

_____   61. Trans means
            (a)   four.
            (b)   green.
            (c)   far away.
            (d)   across.

_____   62. Leuko means
            (a)   blood disease.
            (b)   white.
            (c)   yellow.
            (d)   middle.

_____ 63. Erythro means
    (a) outside of.
    (b) cause.
    (c) red.
    (d) four.

_____ 64. De means
    (a) from, remove.
    (b) double, two.
    (c) difficult, painful.
    (d) too much.

_____ 65. Mega means
    (a) exceptionally small.
    (b) exceptionally large.
    (c) exceptionally short.
    (d) exceptionally tall.

_____ 66. Gyne means
    (a) behind.
    (b) man.
    (c) woman.
    (d) sugar.

_____ 67. Gluc means
    (a) woman.
    (b) around.
    (c) sweet, sugar.
    (d) behind.

_____ 68. Pre means
    (a) new.
    (b) after.
    (c) under.
    (d) before.

_____ 69. Post means
    (a) before.
    (b) after.
    (c) beside.
    (d) behind.

_____   70.   Narc means
(a)   drug.
(b)   night.
(c)   sleep.
(d)   death.

_____   71.   Mal means
(a)   bad.
(b)   good.
(c)   normal.
(d)   black.

_____   72.   Amphi means
(a)   air.
(b)   without.
(c)   near to.
(d)   both sides.

_____   73.   Crypt means
(a)   grave.
(b)   hidden.
(c)   beneath.
(d)   death.

_____   74.   Acro means
(a)   height.
(b)   large.
(c)   both.
(d)   near to.

_____   75.   Ipsi means
(a)   self.
(b)   same.
(c)   slow.
(d)   different.

_____   76.   Hydro means
(a)   half.
(b)   too much.
(c)   water.
(d)   different.

_____ 77. Levo means
    (a) thin.
    (b) white.
    (c) side.
    (d) left.

_____ 78. Postero means
    (a) behind.
    (b) fever.
    (c) backward.
    (d) beside.

_____ 79. Pyro means
    (a) fever.
    (b) pus.
    (c) disease.
    (d) near.

_____ 80. Lipo means
    (a) stone.
    (b) left.
    (c) fat.
    (d) thin.

SUFFERING
SUFFIXES

4

A suffix is a syllable or combination of letters found at the end of a word that adds to the meaning of the word. When defining a word, the suffix is the first definition used. *Note:* Several syllables used here as suffixes are attached to root or stem words for ease in learning the suffixes themselves. There are also a few root words, such as *gram* and *graph*, that are normally used as the final syllable in a word and so are included in this chapter.

SUFFIXES WITH MEANING AND WORD EXAMPLE(S)

DIAGNOSTIC/SYMPTOMATIC TERMS

Suffix	Meaning	Word Example(s)
al	pertaining to, of	beneficial, intercostal, autobiographical
algia	of pain, process, presence or condition of pain	neuralgia
ate	to become	corporate
cele	swelling, hernia, protrusion	cystocele
duct	to lead (also a root word meaning tube)	oviduct, abduct

DIAGNOSTIC/SYMPTOMATIC TERMS

Suffix	Meaning	Word Example(s)
dyne	pain	anodyne
dynia	process, presence, condition of pain	cardiodynia
ectop(y)	displacement, malposition (*ec*= out of; *topy*= place), especially congenital, or present from time of birth	splenectopy
ectopic	of being out of place	ectopic pregnancy
eme(sis)	process/act of vomiting	hematemesis, emetic
em(ia)	presence, process, condition of the blood	anemia, hypoglycemia
ens	of, belonging to	*Homo sapiens*
eum	a place where	museum
form	resembling, shaped	uniform
ful	full of	wonderful
gen(e)	cause, produce	antigen, antipyrogen, genesis
genic	of a cause or production, causing, producing, caused, produced	pathogenic, psychogenic, cardiogenic
gram	instrument that records lines or drawings, instrument making a record	cardiogram, electroencephalogram
graph	lines, drawings, writing, a recording or record	cardiograph, telegraph
ia	process, condition, presence of	anesthesia, proteinuria
iasis	act/process of the process, condition, presence of	lithiasis
ic	of	thoracic
id	morbid (unhealthy, unwholesome) condition of	rabid
ism	process	phototropism
itis	inflammation or infection of	endocarditis, hepatitis
lepsy	seizure	narcolepsy
logy	science, study of	psychology
malacia	process, condition or presence of morbid softening /softness of body part; morbid craving for highly spiced foods	osteomalacia

DIAGNOSTIC/SYMPTOMATIC TERMS

Suffix	Meaning	Word Example(s)
metry	measurement	telemetry
mit	sent, send	transmit, submit
oda, odes	similar to, like, a resemblance	electrodes
oid	resembling form, resembling	keloid, ovoid, android
ology	study of, science	histology
oma	growth, tumor	hepatoma, carcinoma
oncos	tumor, mass, swelling	oncology
os	mouth-like opening or mouth	ileostomy
osis	morbid process or condition, act of, disease	diagnosis, prognosis
ous	of, having	subcutaneous
parous	bearing, giving birth to	multiparous
partum	birth, delivery	postpartum
pathy	disease, suffering	neuropathy
penia	process, condition, presence of too few	leukocytopenia
phag(o)	swallow, eat	aphagia, phagocytosis
phasia	process, condition, presence of speech	aphasia
phobia	process, condition, presence of abnormal fear or dread	photophobia
phoresis	process/act of carrying, bearing, transmission	diaphoresis
phyll	leaf	chlorophyll
plasm	anything formed	ectoplasm
plast	anything formed	neoplast
pnea	breath, breathing	apnea, dyspnea, orthopnea
ptosis	process/act of dropping of an organ (abnormal displacement)	proctoptosis
ptysis	process/act of spitting or saliva	hemoptysis
rrhage	bursting forth	hemorrhage
rrhagia	process, condition, act of bursting forth	metrorrhagia

DIAGNOSTIC/SYMPTOMATIC TERMS

Suffix	Meaning	Word Example(s)
rrhea	flow	rrhea, pyorrhea, dysmenorrhea
rrhexis	process/act of breaking, rupturing	enterorrhexis, cardiorrhexis
scler(o)	hard, hardening	arteriosclerosis, sclerotic
scope	instrument to examine	microscope, proctoscope
scopy	examine, observation, to examine	endoscopy, laparoscopy
sis	process/act of	uresis
spasm	involuntary muscular act, convulsion, twitching, tic	neurospasm
spire	breath or breathing	respiration, inspire
stalsis	process/act of constriction, compression	peristalsis
stasis	process/act of standing, pooling, stagnation (refers to blood)	hemostasis
staxis	process/act of dropping, fall in drops	epistaxis
stom(a)	opening into, a mouth, artificial opening	astomia
tax(o)	arrangement, arrange, order	taxonomy
taxi(s)	arrangement, arrange, order	taxidermist
tic	of, belonging to (also root for spasm)	lunatic, orthotic, opisthotic
trophy	nourishment	atrophy
tropic	of turning toward, tending to turn or change	phototropic, inotropic
tropism	act of turning toward, tending to turn or change; also proper term for growth response stimulus	phototropism
ulous	full of or characterized by	tremulous
uria	process, condition, or presence of the urine	hematuria

SIZE TERMS

Suffix	Meaning	Word Example(s)
cle	small	cuticle, corpuscle
cule	small	molecule
icle	small, little	testicle, icicle, popsicle
ium	small	pericardium
megaly	of or pertaining to abnormal or exceptional enlargement	cardiomegaly
ola	small	arteriola
ole	small	vacuole
ule	small	granule
ulum	small	ovulum
ulus	small	homunculus

TREATMENT, REPAIR, OR SURGICAL TERMS

Suffix	Meaning	Word Example(s)
centesis	puncture of and withdrawal of fluid (process/act of)	pneumocentesis
cise	cut	excise, incision
desis	process/act of binding	arthrodesis
ecta(sis)	extension (process/act of), dilation	bronchiectasis, angiectasis
ectomy	surgical removal of	appendectomy, cholecystectomy
esthes(ia)	process, condition, presence of sensation/feeling	anesthesia, cryesthesia
ize	free from, away, remove, cleanse	cauterize, catheterize
lysis	process/act of dissolution, destruction, decomposition, dissolution, gradual abatement/lessening of disease symptoms	electrolysis, hemodialysis
lytic	belonging to, of, pertaining to dissolution, destruction, gradual abatement, lessening of symptoms of disease	biolytic

Suffix	Meaning	Word Example(s)
ostomy	mouth-like opening (os)/incision formed for drainage	colostomy, tracheostomy
otomy	incision, cutting	tracheotomy, myringotomy
pexy	surgical fixation	mastopexy, hysteropexy
plasty	repair, molding, forming	rhinoplasty
rrhaphy	suture, repair	herniorrhaphy
tomy	cutting, incision	laparotomy, episiotomy

MISCELLANEOUS TERMS*

Suffix	Meaning	Word Example(s)
archy	rule	anarchy
cide	kill	suicide, homicide
cyt(o)	cell	cytomegaly, cytology
cyte	cell	leucocyte, erythrocyte
ist	one who	dermatologist, oncologist
lith(o)	stone	cholelithiasis, lithograph
ped	foot/feet (Latin)	pedal, biped
ped	child (Greek)	pedology, pedophilia
pedia	process, condition, presence of education/children	encyclopedia, pediatrician
pod	foot/feet	orthopod, pseudopod
sophy	wisdom, art, skill	philosophy

*Most of these are root words.

1. SUFFIX DEFINITION EXERCISE

In this exercise, you are given a defined medical term. Define the suffix and then the entire word in the blank, remembering you define the suffix(es) first, then the prefix(es) and root(s). Break each word carefully, making sure you find all the word parts in it. An example is: Luna = moon. Lunatic = of or belonging to the moon.

1.   Neur = nerve. Neuralgia = _____.

2.   An = without or lack of. Anarchy = _____.

3.   Hydro = water/water-like fluid. Hydrocele = _____.

4.   Pneumo = lung. Pneumocentesis = _____.

5.   Patri = father. Patricide = _____.

6.   Ex = outside, away. Excise = _____.

7.   Cuti = skin. Cuticle = _____.

8.   Ovi = ovum or egg. Oviduct = _____.

9.   Ab = from, away. Abduct = _____.

10.   Cardio = heart. Cardiodynia = _____.

11.   Oophor = ovary. Oophorectomy = _____.

12.   Hemat = blood. Hematemesis = _____.

13.   Hypo = under, low, too little. Hypoglycemia = _____.

14.   An = without. Anesthesia = _____.

15. Patho = disease. Pathogenic = _____.

16. Photo = light. Photophobia = _____.

17. Cardio = heart. Cardiograph = _____.

18. Lith = stone. Lithiasis = _____.

19. Arthro = joint. Arthrodesis = _____.

20. Endo = within; card = heart. Endocarditis = _____.

21. Peri = around; card = heart. Pericardium = _____.

22. Narco = sleep. Narcolepsy = _____.

23. Chole = gall or bile. Cholelithiasis = _____.

24. Bio = life. Biology = _____.

25. Cardio = heart. Cardiomegaly = _____.

26. Tele = far away. Telemetry = _____.

27. Trans = across, through, beyond. Transmit = _____.

28. Andro = man. Android = _____.

29. Histo = tissue. Histology = _____.

30. Hepat = liver. Hepatoma = _____.

31. Trache(o) = trachea, or windpipe. Tracheostomy = _____.

32. Multi = many. Multiparous = _____.

33. Neuro = nerve. Neuropathy = _____.

34.   Ortho = straight. Orthopedics = _____.

35.   Leuko = white; cyto = cell. Leukocytopenia = _____.

36.   Figure this one: Phagocytosis = _____.

37.   Mast = breast. Mastopexy = _____.

38.   A = without, from, away. Aphasia = _____.

39.   Pyo = pus. Pyogenic = _____.

40.   Hydro = water, water-like fluid. Hydrophobia = _____.

41.   Chloro = green. Chlorophyll = _____.

42.   Neo = new. Neoplasm = _____.

43.   Rhino = nose. Rhinoplasty = _____.

44.   Dys = difficult, painful. Dyspnea = _____.

45.   Pseudo = false. Pseudopod = _____.

46.   Procto = rectum. Proctoptosis = _____.

47.   Hemo = blood. Hemoptysis = _____.

48.   Colo = colon, or large intestine. Colostomy = _____.

49.   Dys = difficult, painful; meno = menses, menstruation. Dysmenorrhea =

      _____.

50.   Hernio = hernia or rupture. Herniorrhaphy = _____.

51.   Arterio = artery. Arteriosclerosis = _____.

52. Micro = small. A microscope is _____.

53. Endo = inner, inside, within, inward. Endoscopy = _____.

54. Ur(e) = urine. Uresis = _____.

55. Ex = outside, out, away. Expire = _____.

56. Cardio = heart. Cardiodynia = _____.

57. Peri = around. Peristalsis = _____.

58. Taxi(s) = arrangement, arrange, order; derm = skin. Taxidermist =

    _____.

59. Lapar(o) = loins or abdomen. Laparotomy = _____.

60. Atrophy = _____.

61. Ino = within. Inotropic = _____.

62. Hematuria = _____.

63. Lymph = colorless, mostly water, body fluid or part of the lymphatic

    system. Lymphoma = _____.

64. Append = appendix or outgrowth. Appendectomy = _____.

65. Psycho = mind. Psychogenic = _____.

66. Sep(t) = rotten, putrid, disease-causing organisms, or bacteria.

    Septicemia = _____.

67. Pneumo = lung or air. Pneumocentesis = _____.

68. Hepat(o) = liver. Hepatomegaly = _____.

69. Masto = breast. Mastoplasty = _____.

70. Nost = return home or to the familiar. Nostalgia = _____.

71. Psychosis = _____.

72. Auto = self; bio = life; graph = lines, drawings, or writing. Auto-
biographical = _____.

73. Encephalo = brain. Encephalitis = _____.

74. Splen = spleen. Splenectopy = _____.

75. Uni = one. Uniform = _____.

76. Encephalo = brain. Encephalogram = _____.

77. Osteo = bone. Osteomalacia = _____.

78. Dia = across, through, between, completely. Diaphoresis = _____

_____.

79. Anti = against. An antigen is _____.

80. An ectopic pregnancy is _____.

81. Hemo = blood. Hemorrhage = _____.

82. Luna = moon. Lunatic = _____.

83. Electro = electricity. Electrolysis = _____.

84. Neuro = nerve. Neurospasm = _____.

85.   Tremor = a shaking or tremor. Tremulous = _____ .

86.   Mole = mass. Molecule = _____ .

87.   Angi = vessel. Angiectasis = _____ .

88.   A = from, without, away. Astomia = _____ .

89.   Cyte = cell. Erythrocyte = _____ .

90.   Pedograph = _____ .

2. SUFFIX MATCHING EXERCISE

Match the following definitions and suffixes.

_____	1.	condition of abnormal fear/dread of	a. taxo
_____	2.	process/act of	b. stalsis
_____	3.	anything formed	c. pedia
_____	4.	arrangement	d. phobia
_____	5.	free from, away, remove, cleanse	e. id
_____	6.	breath, breathing	f. tomy
_____	7.	breath, breathing	g. scopy
_____	8.	bursting forth	h. cise
_____	9.	condition of	i. plast
_____	10.	condition of	j. pathy
_____	11.	condition of the blood	k. ful
_____	12.	constriction, compression	l. ptosis
_____	13.	cut	m. rrhaphy
_____	14.	cutting, incision	n. spire
_____	15.	condition of sensation or feeling	o. rrhea
_____	16.	disease, suffering	p. osis
_____	17.	displacement, malposition	q. rrhage
_____	18.	act/process of dropping of an organ	r. pod
_____	19.	process, condition, presence of children	s. esthesia
_____	20.	exceptional, abnormal enlargement	t. sis
_____	21.	examine, observation, to examine	u. emia
_____	22.	flow	v. pnea
_____	23.	foot	w. ectopy
_____	24.	suture, repair	x. megaly
_____	25.	full of	y. ize

3. SUFFIX FINDING AND MATCHING EXERCISE

Match definition on the left with the correct italicized suffix in the words on the right.

_____	1.	growth, tumor	a.	ov*oid*
_____	2.	inflammation	b.	arterio*sclerotic*
_____	3.	process, condition, presence in the urine	c.	rhino*plasty*
_____	4.	morbid process, condition	d.	procto*ptosis*
_____	5.	resembling	e.	sui*cide*
_____	6.	disease	f.	hepat*oma*
_____	7.	cause, produce	g.	py*orrhea*
_____	8.	vomiting	h.	a*phagia*
_____	9.	process, condition, presence of too few	i.	laparo*scopy*
_____	10.	swallowing	j.	endocard*itis*
_____	11.	repair	k.	ex*cise*
_____	12.	breathing	l.	ortho*pnea*
_____	13.	act/process of dropping of an organ	m.	hemat*uria*
_____	14.	spitting, saliva	n.	cysto*cele*
_____	15.	bursting forth	o.	leukocyto*penia*
_____	16.	flow	p.	hemo*ptysis*
_____	17.	condition of abnormal fear of	q.	colo*stomy*
_____	18.	repair, molding, forming	r.	neuro*pathy*
_____	19.	hard, hardening	s.	photo*phobia*
_____	20.	examination	t.	an*odyne*
_____	21.	mouth-like opening formed for drainage	u.	diagn*osis*
_____	22.	incision	v.	hemat*emesis*
_____	23.	pain	w.	hemo*rrhage*
_____	24.	swelling, hernia	x.	trache*otomy*
_____	25.	kill	y.	hernio*rrhaphy*
_____	26.	cut	z.	anti*gen*

4. SUFFIX FINDING AND MATCHING EXERCISE

Match definition on the left with the correct italicized suffix in the words on the right.

_____	1.	of process, condition of pain	a.	encephalo*graph*
_____	2.	surgical removal of	b.	narco*lepsy*
_____	3.	process, presence, condition of the blood	c.	leuko*cyte*
_____	4.	a record	d.	cholelith*iasis*
_____	5.	instrument recording lines or drawings	e.	hemi*esthesia*
_____	6.	away, remove, free from	f.	osteo*malacia*
_____	7.	seizure	g.	peri*stalsis*
_____	8.	study of, science	h.	ab*duct*
_____	9.	of receding of disease symptoms	i.	*ped*ophilia
_____	10.	sensation, feeling	j.	neur*algia*
_____	11.	pertaining to, of	k.	angi*ectasis*
_____	12.	of a cause or production	l.	mon*archy*
_____	13.	act of puncture and withdrawal of fluid	m.	hypo*glycemia*
_____	14.	condition of morbid softening	n.	proct*ology*
_____	15.	cell	o.	inter*costal*
_____	16.	process of extension, dilation	p.	hystero*pexy*
_____	17.	nourishment	q.	cauter*ize*
_____	18.	process of, presence of	r.	carcino*genic*
_____	19.	surgical fixation	s.	append*ectomy*
_____	20.	child	t.	laparo*scope*
_____	21.	to lead	u.	cardio*megaly*
_____	22.	instrument to examine	v.	pericard*ium*
_____	23.	small	w.	a*trophy*
_____	24.	rule	x.	electrocardio*gram*
_____	25.	exceptional enlargement	y.	thora*centesis*
_____	26.	act of constriction, compression	z.	bio*lytic*

5. SUFFIX PUZZLE

ACROSS

1. Spitting, saliva
3. Examine
5. The Boy King
6. Condition of blood
9. Small
11. Hard
13. Note after "fa"
14. Hard
18. Foot
21. What one rows with
23. Turning
24. Produced by, producing
25. Swallowing, eating
26. Masculine pronoun
27. Membership fee
28. Nickname for Edward
29. Process, condition
31. Tree fluid
33. Cut
34. Greek letter
36. Receding of disease symptoms
38. Too few
39. English "bye"
42. Flow
44. X-___
45. Mouth-like-opening formed for drainage
49. Cutting, incising
52. Lines, drawings
54. One who taps
55. Honey ___
56. It stinks (abbr.)
57. Pain
58. Small
59. Actress ___ West
61. Record
62. Animal foot
63. Small
65. Swelling, hernia
69. Away, remove, free from
70. Study of, science
72. What makes breads rise (plural)
75. Margarine
77. To become
78. Presence of in the urine
79. Anything formed
81. Arrangement
83. Tear
84. What ___ is it?
85. Please eat oranges (abbr.)
86. South Yorkshire (abbr.)

DOWN

2. Pronoun
4. Small
5. Turning
6. Sensation, feeling
7. ___ or less
8. Cleo's snake
9. ___ else
10. Study of, science
12. Dogs have four of these
15. Kill
16. La. State Univ.
17. Vomiting
18. Breathing
19. Resembling
20. Where US capital is
22. Suture, repair
25. Anything formed
30. Inflammation of
32. Repair, form, shape
33. Coney Island (abbr.)
35. Masculine pronoun
37. Instrument to examine
38. Abnormal fear of
40. Pain
41. Growth, tumor
42. Bursting forth
43. Egyptian god
46. Sun ___
47. Military Police (abbr.)
48. Long for
50. Cat's ___
51. Japanese money
53. Small
56. Disease
57. To lead
59. Enlargement
60. Surgical removal
62. Swallow, eat
64. Seizure
66. Small
67. Leaf
68. Dropping of an organ
70. Process, condition
71. Republican Party (abbr.)
73. Arrangement
74. Opening
76. Hearing organ
78. Small
80. Member of Parliament (abbr.)
82. Location

SUFFIX PUZZLE

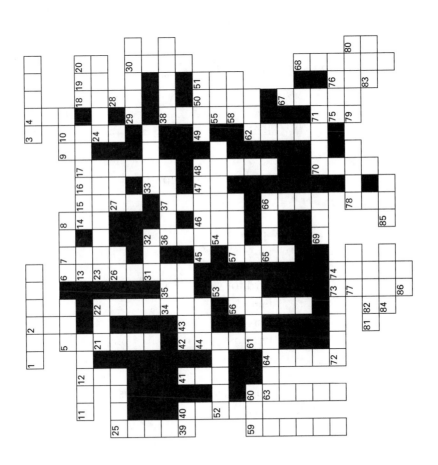

6. SUFFIX MULTIPLE CHOICE EXERCISE

Select the best answer and write the letters of your choice in the space.

_____   1.   The word for constriction is
(a)   emesis.
(b)   iasis.
(c)   rrhexis.
(d)   stalsis.

_____   2.   The word for flow is
(a)   rrhage.
(b)   emesis.
(c)   plast.
(d)   rrhea.

_____   3.   The word for turning toward is
(a)   tropic.
(b)   taxis.
(c)   spire.
(d)   parous.

_____   4.   The word for study of or science is
(a)   logy.
(b)   lysis.
(c)   lepsy.
(d)   lytic.

_____   5.   The word for suture or repair is
(a)   rrhaphy.
(b)   rrhage.
(c)   rrhea.
(d)   rrhexis.

_____   6.   The word for nourishment is
(a)   phobia.
(b)   phasia.
(c)   trophy.
(d)   phago.

_____   7. The word for presence of in the urine is
      (a)   osis.
      (b)   uria.
      (c)   itis.
      (d)   ule.

_____   8. The word for disease is
      (a)   osis.
      (b)   itis.
      (c)   pathy.
      (d)   plasty.

_____   9. The word for incision is
      (a)   ostomy.
      (b)   cise.
      (c)   oda.
      (d)   otomy.

_____   10. The word for mouth-like opening is
      (a)   cele.
      (b)   pexy.
      (c)   ostomy.
      (d)   otomy.

_____   11. The word for morbid process, condition, or disease is
      (a)   ectasis.
      (b)   osis.
      (c)   ectomy.
      (d)   emesis.

_____   12. The word for growth or tumor is
      (a)   pathy.
      (b)   lysis.
      (c)   oma.
      (d)   itis.

_____   13. The word for abnormal enlargement is
      (a)   trophy.
      (b)   spasm.
      (c)   algia.
      (d)   megaly.

_____   14.   The word for free from or remove is

(a)   eum.
(b)   ize.
(c)   phyll.
(d)   rrhexis.

_____   15.   The word for inflammation or infection of is

(a)   itis.
(b)   osis.
(c)   pathy.
(d)   rrhea.

_____   16.   The word for condition of is

(a)   itis.
(b)   id.
(c)   ostomy.
(d)   esthesia.

_____   17.   The word for record is

(a)   gram.
(b)   graph.
(c)   pathy.
(d)   pedia.

_____   18.   The word for produced by is

(a)   uria.
(b)   genic.
(c)   itis.
(d)   osis.

_____   19.   The word for to lead is

(a)   lytic.
(b)   spire.
(c)   duct.
(d)   sis.

_____   20.   The word for condition of the blood is

(a)   rrhage.
(b)   osis.
(c)   iasis.
(d)   emia.

_____   21.   The word for lines or drawings or a record is
                  (a)   graph.
                  (b)   gram.
                  (c)   genic.
                  (d)   gen.

_____   22.   The word for breathing is
                  (a)   pnea.
                  (b)   penia.
                  (c)   cide.
                  (d)   phago.

_____   23.   The word for repair or molding is
                  (a)   lith.
                  (b)   taxis.
                  (c)   plasty.
                  (d)   algia.

_____   24.   The word for process or condition is
                  (a)   oid.
                  (b)   itis.
                  (c)   osis.
                  (d)   iasis.

_____   25.   The word for speech is
                  (a)   phasia.
                  (b)   ptosis.
                  (c)   ptysis.
                  (d)   pexy.

_____   26.   The word for spitting or saliva is
                  (a)   pnea.
                  (b)   ptysis.
                  (c)   ptosis.
                  (d)   ule.

_____   27.   The word for the act of a break or rupture is
                  (a)   rrhea.
                  (b)   rrhexis.
                  (c)   rrhage.
                  (d)   rrhaphy.

_____ 28.   The word for sensation or feeling is
    (a)   ectasis.
    (b)   esthesia.
    (c)   lysis.
    (d)   itis.

_____ 29.   The word for stone is
    (a)   sophy.
    (b)   stoma.
    (c)   lytic.
    (d)   lith.

_____ 30.   The word for surgical removal is
    (a)   ectomy.
    (b)   ectopy.
    (c)   ectasis.
    (d)   emesis.

_____ 31.   The word for surgical fixation is
    (a)   rrhaphy.
    (b)   pexy.
    (c)   tomy.
    (d)   taxis.

_____ 32.   The word for cutting or incision is
    (a)   itis.
    (b)   tomy.
    (c)   osis.
    (d)   ptosis.

_____ 33.   The word for vomiting is
    (a)   itis.
    (b)   centesis.
    (c)   emesis.
    (d)   lepsy.

_____ 34.   The word for pain or of pain is
    (a)   duct.
    (b)   dynia.
    (c)   archy.
    (d)   algia.

_____ 35. The word for binding is
    (a) otomy.
    (b) desis.
    (c) centesis.
    (d) uria.

_____ 36. The word for an instrument to examine is
    (a) metry.
    (b) scopy.
    (c) scope.
    (d) taxis.

_____ 37. The word for belonging to is
    (a) archy.
    (b) tic.
    (c) lepsy.
    (d) ptosis.

_____ 38. The word for bursting forth is
    (a) lysis.
    (b) rrhage.
    (c) rrhea.
    (d) rrhexis.

_____ 39. The word for dropping of an organ is
    (a) rrhaphy.
    (b) plasty.
    (c) ptosis.
    (d) ptysis.

_____ 40. The word for swallowing or eating is
    (a) osis.
    (b) oma.
    (c) stomy.
    (d) phag.

_____ 41. The word for too few is
    (a) pedia.
    (b) pnea.
    (c) penia.
    (d) phoresis.

_____ 42. The word for swelling or hernia is
     (a) sclero.
     (b) cele.
     (c) pathy.
     (d) oma.

_____ 43. The word for abnormal fear or dread is
     (a) phobia.
     (b) algia.
     (c) dynia.
     (d) phasia.

_____ 44. The word for destruction is
     (a) centesis.
     (b) itis.
     (c) osis.
     (d) lysis.

_____ 45. The word for measurement is
     (a) penia.
     (b) megaly.
     (c) metry.
     (d) ostomy.

_____ 46. The word for kill is
     (a) necro.
     (b) cele.
     (c) cide.
     (d) cise.

_____ 47. The word for full of is
     (a) ful.
     (b) cle.
     (c) eum.
     (d) osis.

_____ 48. The word for opening or mouth is
     (a) itis.
     (b) phyll.
     (c) os.
     (d) ful.

_____   49.   The word for produce is

    (a)   gen.

    (b)   cle.

    (c)   parous.

    (d)   plasty.

_____   50.   The word for cut is

    (a)   emia.

    (b)   ectopy.

    (c)   excise.

    (d)   cise.

GETTING DOWN TO
ROOTS
5

The root or stem is the main body or basic component of a word. Several roots or stems have been used in previous chapters with appropriate prefixes and/or suffixes attached but are reviewed in this chapter. With the exception of sexual organs, all organs and body parts shown in the figure of the man are also found in the woman, and vice-versa. Although *neuro* (nerve) is shown in the male head, nerves are found in all parts of the body; the same holds true for *myo* (muscle), *osteo* (bone), *arthro* (joint), *arterio* (artery), *phlebo* (vein), and so on. Also, only one of each organ is shown, although there are many organs with two or more of each—two eyes, ears, ovaries, more than one tooth, and so on. These drawings will provide a general idea of the location of an organ. By using the imaginary lines from Chapter 3, you can also identify the quadrant in which a particular organ is located.

ROOTS WITH MEANING AND WORD EXAMPLE(S)

ORGANS OR BODY COMPONENTS SHOWN IN THE MALE (*ANDRO*) DRAWING

Root	Meaning	Word Example(s)
arteri(o)	artery	arteriogram, arteritis
arthr(o)	joint	arthritis, arthrodesis
card(i)(io)	heart	endocarditis, cardiopathy

Root	Meaning	Word Example(s)
cephal(o)	head	hydrocephalus, bicephalic
chondr(o)	cartilage	chondroma
coccyx	last bone of spine—tailbone	coccygodynia, sacrocoxitis
cost(o)	rib	intercostal
cyst(o)	sac, bladder	cystoscopy, cholecystectomy
encephal(o)	brain (within the head)	encephalitis
ili(o)	ilium, large pelvic bone	iliolumbar, iliac
lapar(o)	abdomen, loins	laparotomy
my(o)	muscle	endomyocarditis
myel(o)	spinal cord or bone marrow	myelogram, osteomyelitis
nas(o)	nose	nasogastric tube
nephr(o)	kidney	nephritis, nephrologist
neur(o)	nerve	neurogenic, neoropathy
or(o,a,i)	an opening or mouth	oral, orad
orch(i,o,id)	testicle	orchi(d)ectomy, cryptorchi(d)ism
oste(o)	bone	osteoarthritis, osteomyoma
phleb(o)	vein	phlebitis, phlebotomist
pleur(o)	rib, pleura, side	pleuritis
pleura	membrane lining walls of chest cavity	pleursy
prostat(o)	prostate	prostatitis, prostatic
pyel(o)	kidney pelvis	pyelogram, pyelitis
rachi(o)	spine	rachicentesis, rachigraph
rachis	column of vertebrae in the spine, vertebral column	
ren(i,o)	kidney	renipelvic, renopathy
rhin(o)	nose	rhinorrhea, rhinoplasty
sacr(o)	sacrum, below lumbar spine, above coccyx	sacroiliac, sacral
stern(o)	sternum, breast bone	sternocostal, sternotomy
stomat(o)	mouth	stomatitis, stomatomalacia
thorac(o)	chest, thorax, or pleural cavity	pneumothorax, thoracentesis
thyr(o)	thyroid gland	thyroadenitis, thyromegaly
ureter(o)	ureter	ureterectomy

ORGANS OR BODY COMPONENTS SHOWN IN THE FEMALE
(*GYN/E/EC/ECO*) DRAWING

Root	Meaning	Word Example(s)
an(o)	anus (last part of colon)	anal, anosigmoidoscopy, anorectum
append	appendix	appendectomy
bronch(o)	bronchus	bronchitis, bronchogenic
cholecyst(o)	gall or bile bladder	cholecystectomy
choledoch(o)	gall or bile tube or duct	choledocholithiasis
col(o)	colon or large intestine	colitis, colectomy
colp(o)	vagina	colporrhaphy, colpitis
crani(o)	skull	craniotomy
cut(i)	skin	cuticle
cutane	skin	subcutaneous
dent(i,o)	tooth/teeth	dentist
dont	tooth/teeth	orthodontist
derm(a,at)	skin	dermatitis, scleroderma
enter(o)	intestine, small intestine	enteritis, gastroenteritis
esophag(o)	esophagus	esophagitis, esophagectasia
gastr(o)	stomach	hemigastrectomy, gastritis
gloss(o)	tongue	glossitis, glossary
hepa(t,to)	liver	hepatitis, hepatomegaly
hyster(o)	uterus	oophorohysterectomy
ile(o)	ileum, distal part of small intestine	ileitis
lingu(o)	tongue	bilingual, linguistics
mast(o)	breast	mastectomy, gynecomastia
metr(o)	uterus	metrorrhagia
ocul(o)	eye	oculist
oophor(o)	ovary	oophorectomy
ophthalm(o)	eye	ophthalmologist
ot(o)	ear	otalgia, otitis, otology
pancre	secretes fluids, like insulin	pancreatic, pancreatolithectomy
pharyng(o)	pharynx	pharyngitis
pleura	membrane lining walls of chest cavity	pleuralgia
pneum(o)	lung, air	pneumonitis, pneumatic tire
proct(o)	rectum	proctoscope

Root	Meaning	Word Example(s)
salping(o)	tube, oviduct or eustachian tube	salpingogram
splen(o)	spleen	splenectopy
trache(o)	trachea	tracheotomy
uter(o)	uterus	uterogenic
womb	uterus	womb

ORGANS OR BODY COMPONENTS NOT SHOWN IN DRAWINGS

Root	Meaning	Word Example(s)
aden(o)	gland	adenopathy, adenoid
angi(o)	vessel	angiogram, angiectasis
blephar(o)	eyelid or eyelash	blepharoplasty, blepharectomy
chil(o)	lip	lipochilectomy
cili(a,o)	small hair, eyelash, or lid	ciliectomy
colpos	vaginal mouth/cervix	colposcopy
corpus	body	corpuscle
cyt(o)	cell	cytology
cyte	cell	erythrocyte
doch(o)	duct	choledocholithosis
fibr(o)	connective tissue	fibrolipoma, fibroplasia
hem(a,o)	blood	hemopathy, hematuria
hemat(o)	blood	hematocytopenia
hist(o)	tissue	histogram
kerat(o)	cornea, horn-like	radial keratotomy, keratodermia, keratosis
meninges	membranes over brain and spinal cord	meningitis
myring(o)	tympanic membrane/eardrum	myringotomy
onych(o)	nail, claw	schizonychia, epionychial
onco(s)	tumor	oncology
op(t,tic)	(of, belonging to) eye	optician
or(a)	mouth	oral, orad
os	mouth	tracheostomy
otic	of the ear	otic
ped/pœd (Latin)	foot	pedal, orthop(œ)edics, pedograph
pleur(o)	pleura, rib, side	pleuritis
pod	foot	quadrapod

Root	Meaning	Word Example(s)
poie	making	hematopoiesis
rachia	of spinal fluid	rachicentesis
rachis	column of vertebrae in the spine	spine rachialgia
renal	of or pertaining to the kidney	adrenal
stomach	stomach (gastro)	stomachalgia
vas(o)	vessel, blood vessel, or duct	vasoconstriction, vasectomy, vascular

MISCELLANEOUS ROOTS

Root	Meaning	Word Example(s)
ambul	walk	ambulate
carcin(o)	cancer	carcinogenic, carcinoma
chole	bile, gall	cholecystic
chrom(a,at,o)	color	monochrome, chromatopsia
cry(o)	freeze, cold	cryesthesia
cysto	sac or bladder	cystoscopy, cystitis
glob(o)	ball, globe	hemoglobin
lip(o)	fat	liposuction, myolipoma
lith(o)	stone	cholelithiasis, nephrolithectomy, lithograph
men(o)	menses	dysmenorrhea, amenorrhea
muc(o)	mucus	mucocele, mucoid
myco	fungus	mycology
olig(o)	few, scanty	oliguria
peps	digest or cook	dyspepsia
thrombo	clot	thrombocytopenia

DRAWING OF THE MAN

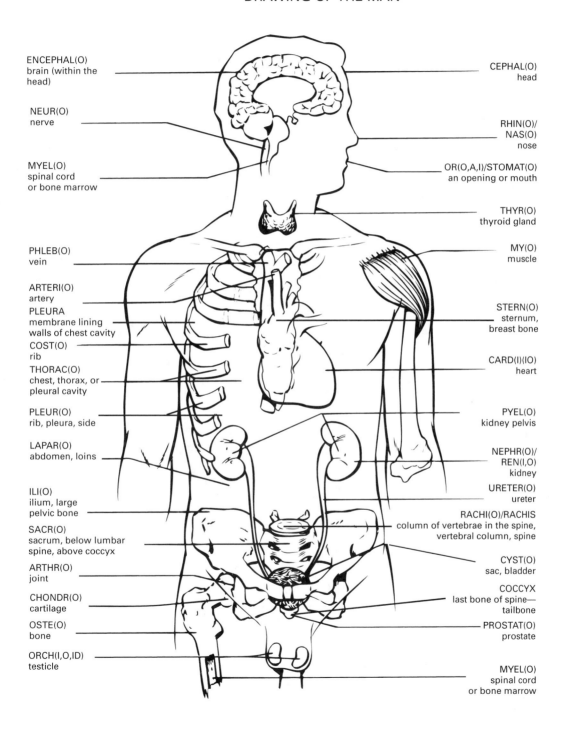

ENCEPHAL(O)
brain (within the
head)

NEUR(O)
nerve

MYEL(O)
spinal cord
or bone marrow

PHLEB(O)
vein

ARTERI(O)
artery

PLEURA
membrane lining
walls of chest cavity

COST(O)
rib

THORAC(O)
chest, thorax, or
pleural cavity

PLEUR(O)
rib, pleura, side

LAPAR(O)
abdomen, loins

ILI(O)
ilium, large
pelvic bone

SACR(O)
sacrum, below lumbar
spine, above coccyx

ARTHR(O)
joint

CHONDR(O)
cartilage

OSTE(O)
bone

ORCH(I,O,ID)
testicle

CEPHAL(O)
head

RHIN(O)/
NAS(O)
nose

OR(O,A,I)/STOMAT(O)
an opening or mouth

THYR(O)
thyroid gland

MY(O)
muscle

STERN(O)
sternum,
breast bone

CARD(I)(IO)
heart

PYEL(O)
kidney pelvis

NEPHR(O)/
REN(I,O)
kidney

URETER(O)
ureter

RACHI(O)/RACHIS
column of vertebrae in the spine,
vertebral column, spine

CYST(O)
sac, bladder

COCCYX
last bone of spine—
tailbone

PROSTAT(O)
prostate

MYEL(O)
spinal cord
or bone marrow

DRAWING OF THE WOMAN

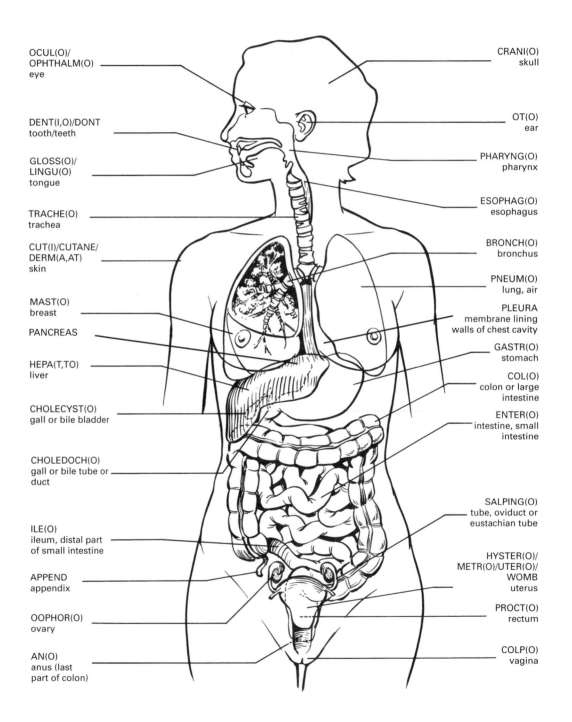

OCUL(O)/
OPHTHALM(O)
eye

DENT(I,O)/DONT
tooth/teeth

GLOSS(O)/
LINGU(O)
tongue

TRACHE(O)
trachea

CUT(I)/CUTANE/
DERM(A,AT)
skin

MAST(O)
breast

PANCREAS

HEPA(T,TO)
liver

CHOLECYST(O)
gall or bile bladder

CHOLEDOCH(O)
gall or bile tube or
duct

ILE(O)
ileum, distal part
of small intestine

APPEND
appendix

OOPHOR(O)
ovary

AN(O)
anus (last
part of colon)

CRANI(O)
skull

OT(O)
ear

PHARYNG(O)
pharynx

ESOPHAG(O)
esophagus

BRONCH(O)
bronchus

PNEUM(O)
lung, air

PLEURA
membrane lining
walls of chest cavity

GASTR(O)
stomach

COL(O)
colon or large
intestine

ENTER(O)
intestine, small
intestine

SALPING(O)
tube, oviduct or
eustachian tube

HYSTER(O)/
METR(O)/UTER(O)/
WOMB
uterus

PROCT(O)
rectum

COLP(O)
vagina

1. INTERNAL ORGAN MATCHING EXERCISE

The terms on the left pertain to internal organs. Match the root on the left with the correct definition on the right, placing the letter in the space provided.

_____	1.	cardio	a.	joint
_____	2.	gastro	b.	eardrum
_____	3.	myelo	c.	brain
_____	4.	cholecysto	d.	large pelvic bone
_____	5.	nephro	e.	membrane lining chest walls
_____	6.	procto	f.	bone marrow/spinal cord
_____	7.	myringo	g.	heart
_____	8.	salpingo	h.	gland
_____	9.	broncho	i.	fallopian tube
_____	10.	ilio	j.	small intestine
_____	11.	hepato	k.	gallbladder
_____	12.	arthro	l.	artery
_____	13.	pyelo	m.	kidney
_____	14.	ileo	n.	bone
_____	15.	costo	o.	liver
_____	16.	neuro	p.	vein
_____	17.	pleura	q.	pelvis of kidney
_____	18.	oophoro	r.	last part of small intestine
_____	19.	encephalo	s.	bronchus
_____	20.	osteo	t.	nerve
_____	21.	adeno	u.	stomach
_____	22.	phlebo	v.	ovary
_____	23.	orchio	w.	rectum
_____	24.	entero	x.	rib
_____	25.	arterio	y.	testis

2. ROOT MULTIPLE CHOICE EXERCISE

Select the correct answer(s) and write the letter(s) of your choice in the space.

_____   1.   Adeno is the root for
   (a)   vessel.
   (b)   man.
   (c)   gland.
   (d)   all of the above
   (e)   none of the above

_____   2.   The root(s) for liver is/are
   (a)   hemato.
   (b)   hepato.
   (c)   colpo.
   (d)   all of the above
   (e)   none of the above

_____   3.   Nas is the root for
   (a)   nose.
   (b)   nerve.
   (c)   kidney.
   (d)   all of the above
   (e)   none of the above

_____   4.   Optic is the root for
   (a)   nerve.
   (b)   eye.
   (c)   ovary.
   (d)   mouth.
   (e)   none of the above

_____   5.   The root(s) for stone is/are
   (a)   rocko.
   (b)   litho.
   (c)   lipo.
   (d)   linguo.
   (e)   stomato.

_____   6. Cili is the root for
        (a)   small hair or eyelash.
        (b)   dish made with peppers.
        (c)   cartilage in joints.
        (d)   lips around the mouth.

_____   7. The proper term(s) for the kidney pelvis is/are
        (a)   pyelo.
        (b)   cysto.
        (c)   procto.
        (d)   neuro.

_____   8. Globo is the root for
        (a)   the world.
        (b)   ball.
        (c)   fat.
        (d)   tongue.

_____   9. The root(s) for foot is/are
        (a)   pod.
        (b)   ped.
        (c)   ortho.
        (d)   pedia.
        (e)   phleb.

_____   10. Andro is/are the root(s) for
        (a)   man.
        (b)   gland.
        (c)   vessel.
        (d)   robot.
        (e)   human.

_____   11. The root word(s) for nerve is/are
        (a)   fibr.
        (b)   angi.
        (c)   nephro.
        (d)   neuro.
        (e)   neo.

_____ 12. Chondro is/are the root(s) for
   (a) joint.
   (b) connective tissue.
   (c) tissue.
   (d) cartilage.
   (e) none of the above

_____ 13. The root(s) for mind is/are
   (a) psycho.
   (b) cephalo.
   (c) pyelo.
   (d) all of the above
   (e) none of the above

_____ 14. The root(s) for fungus is/are
   (a) myco.
   (b) tinea.
   (c) myo.
   (d) all of the above
   (e) none of the above

_____ 15. The root(s) for tongue is/are
   (a) glosso.
   (b) linguo.
   (c) salpingo.
   (d) all of the above
   (e) none of the above

_____ 16. Intercostal means pertaining to between the
   (a) vein.
   (b) chest.
   (c) cartilage.
   (d) all of the above
   (e) none of the above

_____ 17. Pneumo is the root word for
   (a) breast.
   (b) ribs.
   (c) heart.
   (d) lung.
   (e) none of the above

_____   18.   The root(s) for skin is/are
        (a)   cuti.
        (b)   cutane.
        (c)   derm.
        (d)   all of the above
        (e)   none of the above

_____   19.   The root(s) for body is/are
        (a)   andro.
        (b)   corpus.
        (c)   oophor.
        (d)   all of the above
        (e)   none of the above

_____   20.   The root for intestine is
        (a)   colo.
        (b)   gastro.
        (c)   entero.
        (d)   procto.
        (e)   none of the above

_____   21.   Angi is the root for
        (a)   joint.
        (b)   man.
        (c)   vessel.
        (d)   artery.
        (e)   clot.

_____   22.   Thromb is the definition of
        (a)   cut.
        (b)   clot.
        (c)   closure.
        (d)   beat.
        (e)   blood.

_____   23.   The root(s) for tissue is/are
        (a)   histo.
        (b)   cysto.
        (c)   hystero.
        (d)   all of the above
        (e)   none of the above

_____ 24. Gastro is the root for
  (a) colon.
  (b) intestine.
  (c) tongue.
  (d) stomach.
  (e) none of the above

_____ 25. The root(s) for eye is/are
  (a) ocul.
  (b) ophthalmo.
  (c) opti.
  (d) all of the above
  (e) none of the above

_____ 26. The root(s) for bile or gall is/are
  (a) chole.
  (b) sac.
  (c) cele.
  (d) all of the above
  (e) none of the above

_____ 27. The root for child is
  (a) gyne.
  (b) pedia.
  (c) andro.
  (d) all of the above
  (e) none of the above

_____ 28. The root(s) for vein is/are
  (a) thrombo.
  (b) phlebo.
  (c) vaso.
  (d) hemato.
  (e) none of the above

_____ 29. The root(s) for chest is/are
  (a) costo.
  (b) thoraco.
  (c) pleuro.
  (d) pneumo.
  (e) pectoro.

_____   30.   Oste is the root for
     (a)   bone.
     (b)   eye.
     (c)   opening stomach to mouth.
     (d)   mouth.
     (e)   none of the above

_____   31.   Vaso means
     (a)   tube.
     (b)   blood vessel, duct, or vessel.
     (c)   enlargement.
     (d)   urn.
     (e)   vase.

_____   32.   Hyster is the root for
     (a)   tissue.
     (b)   mental illness.
     (c)   womb.
     (d)   all of the above
     (e)   none of the above

_____   33.   The root(s) for cell is/are
     (a)   costo.
     (b)   cyto.
     (c)   cysto.
     (d)   all of the above
     (e)   none of the above

_____   34.   Col is the root for
     (a)   rib.
     (b)   colon.
     (c)   vagina.
     (d)   body.
     (e)   none of the above

_____   35.   The root for bronchus is
     (a)   lapar.
     (b)   linguo.
     (c)   pneumo.
     (d)   all of the above
     (e)   none of the above

_____ 36. Hemat is the root for
    (a)   uterus.
    (b)   tissue.
    (c)   blood.
    (d)   liver.
    (e)   none of the above

_____ 37. Chil is the root for
    (a)   lip.
    (b)   bile.
    (c)   fat.
    (d)   muscle.
    (e)   hypothermia.

_____ 38. The root word(s) for fungus is/are
    (a)   penia.
    (b)   tinea.
    (c)   orchi.
    (d)   all of the above
    (e)   none of the above

_____ 39. Myo is the root for
    (a)   nose.
    (b)   muscle.
    (c)   mucus.
    (d)   all of the above
    (e)   none of the above

_____ 40. The root(s) for horn or cornea is/are
    (a)   hernia.
    (b)   corpus.
    (c)   col.
    (d)   kerato.
    (e)   none of the above

_____   41.   The root(s) for tooth is/are

    (a)   dontist.

    (b)   denti.

    (c)   Dentyne.

    (d)   ortho.

    (e)   none of the above

_____   42.   The root(s) for connective tissue is/are

    (a)   phlebo.

    (b)   fibro.

    (c)   chondro.

    (d)   all of the above

    (e)   none of the above

_____   43.   Cryo is the root for

    (a)   eyelid.

    (b)   sac or bladder.

    (c)   rib cage.

    (d)   freeze.

    (e)   cold.

_____   44.   The root(s) for sac or bladder is/are

    (a)   cysto.

    (b)   colpo.

    (c)   cyto.

    (d)   colo.

    (e)   none of the above

_____   45.   Rachi is

    (a)   an instrument of torture.

    (b)   spine.

    (c)   spinal cord.

    (d)   all of the above

    (e)   none of the above

_____   46.   Thoraco means
(a)   chest.
(b)   breast.
(c)   thyroid.
(d)   all of the above
(e)   none of the above

_____   47.   The word(s) for vertebral column is/are
(a)   rachis.
(b)   rhino.
(c)   renal.
(d)   all of the above
(e)   none of the above

_____   48.   Carcin is the root word for
(a)   colon.
(b)   cancer.
(c)   tumor.
(d)   all of the above
(e)   none of the above

_____   49.   The word(s) for liver is/are
(a)   hepato.
(b)   hystero.
(c)   hemato.
(d)   all of the above
(e)   none of the above

_____   50.   Encephalo means
(a)   within the hair.
(b)   within the skull.
(c)   within the brain.
(d)   all of the above
(e)   none of the above

3. ROOT MATCHING EXERCISE

Match the following in the left column with the definition in the right column.

_____	1.	cranio	a.	menstruation
_____	2.	chromat	b.	stone
_____	3.	kerato	c.	brain
_____	4.	globo	d.	freeze, cold
_____	5.	vaso	e.	bone
_____	6.	linguo	f.	cyto
_____	7.	meno	g.	gland
_____	8.	glosso	h.	mucus
_____	9.	carcino	i.	vein
_____	10.	encephalo	j.	body
_____	11.	gastro	k.	cornea
_____	12.	osteo	l.	fat
_____	13.	entero	m.	skull
_____	14.	phlebo	n.	ball
_____	15.	tooth	o.	vessel
_____	16.	cryo	p.	stomach
_____	17.	corpus	q.	tongue
_____	18.	muco	r.	color
_____	19.	costo	s.	dont
_____	20.	adeno	t.	intestine
_____	21.	chondro	u.	rib
_____	22.	lipo	v.	tongue
_____	23.	pyelo	w.	nephro
_____	24.	kidney	x.	cancer
_____	25.	litho	y.	kidney pelvis
_____	26.	cell	z.	cartilage

4. ROOT PUZZLE

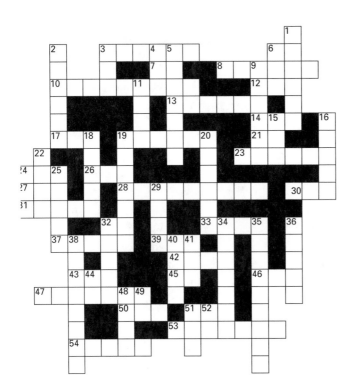

ACROSS

3. Vein
6. J,k,l,_,_,o
7. Noise of a bear
8. Liver
10. Oviduct or eustachian tube
12. Fish egg
13. Kidney
14. Baby or bird noise
17. Mouths
19. Joint
21. English "bye"
23. Body
24. What you kiss with
26. Dine
27. One of *Little Women*
28. Brain
30. Muscle
31. Spinal cord
32. USMC trainer (abbr.)
33. Of the ear
37. Bone
39. Mouth
42. Time measure
43. Biblical character
45. He, she, or __
46. August birth sign
47. Ovary
50. Curvy letter
51. Unruly crowd
53. Eardrum
54. Stomach

DOWN

1. Intestine
2. Stomach
3. "__ goes the weasel"
4. Ovum
5. Bronchus
6. Chairman __
9. Rectal
11. Nerve
15. Used in boat
16. Rib
18. Gland
19. Artery
20. Testicle
22. Covered with frost
24. On the __ (criminal)
25. Renal pelvis
29. Cell
32. Tooth
34. Clots
35. Vessel carrying bile
36. Fat (plural)
38. Oviduct
40. Nose
41. Virginian "out"
44. Word of surprise
48. Why you sleep
49. Mouth
51. Muscle
52. __ else

5. ROOT MATCHING EXERCISE

Match the following left column with the definition in the right column.

_____	1. oligo	a.	gland
_____	2. utero	b.	lip
_____	3. rachi	c.	abdomen
_____	4. rachis	d.	child
_____	5. adeno	e.	anus
_____	6. uretero	f.	foot
_____	7. cysto	g.	thyro
_____	8. thoraco	h.	chest
_____	9. cephalo	i.	gall
_____	10. ano	j.	uterus
_____	11. kerato	k.	vertebral column
_____	12. thrombo	l.	nerve
_____	13. partum	m.	skin
_____	14. coccyx	n.	duct
_____	15. chilo	o.	scanty
_____	16. mast	p.	clot
_____	17. pod	q.	education
_____	18. pedia	r.	breast
_____	19. ped	s.	head
_____	20. chole	t.	bladder
_____	21. thyro	u.	tailbone
_____	22. cilia	v.	birth or delivery
_____	23. cutane	w.	cornea
_____	24. laparo	x.	spine
_____	25. neuro	y.	eyelash
_____	26. docho	z.	ureter

6. ROOT-INTERNAL ORGAN PUZZLE

ACROSS

2. Trachea
4. Bone marrow—spinal cord
7. Lung
8. Appendix
10. Small intestine
11. Liver
13. Chest
17. Internat. Line (abbr.)
19. Yield or grant
20. From, away
22. Spinal cord
23. Nerve
24. Tough nut (abbr.)
25. Vein
28. Esophagus
31. Bile duct
33. Laugh sound
34. Eye
35. Bull fight cheer
37. Mouth
43. Inferior (position)
44. Storage under roof
46. Eustachian tube
48. Brain
51. Mouth
52. Emergency Room (abbr.)
53. Muscle
55. Anus
57. Post Office (abbr.)
58. Spanish gold
61. Nose
62. Joint
63. Alkaline balance
64. Noses
66. Thyroid
68. Writing instrument
69. Large intestine
70. Long period of time
71. Rib
73. Stomach
76. Uterus
77. Eye
79. Tooth
81. Testicles
82. Abdomen
83. Mouth

DOWN

1. Skin
2. A preposition
3. Liver
5. Woman
6. More than one kidney pelvis
8. Artery
9. Rectum
12. Prostate
14. Kidney
15. Near
16. Head
17. Ileum
18. Anus
20. Entirety
21. Honey maker
22. Cow sound
26. Santa says
27. Black dog (abbr.)
29. Ear
30. Tongue
31. Gall bladder
32. Skull
36. Female sheep
37. Sacrum
38. Ovary
39. Over six feet is
40. Ear
41. Bladder
42. Bile duct
43. Bronchus
45. Cartilage
47. Pharynx
49. Kidney
50. Heart
53. Breast
54. Vagina
56. Bile
59. Blood factor
60. Piggy noise
63. Renal pelvis
65. Uterus
67. Know
72. Tattled
74. Of the ear
75. Ilium
78. Man
80. Part of small intestine

INTERNAL ORGAN PUZZLE

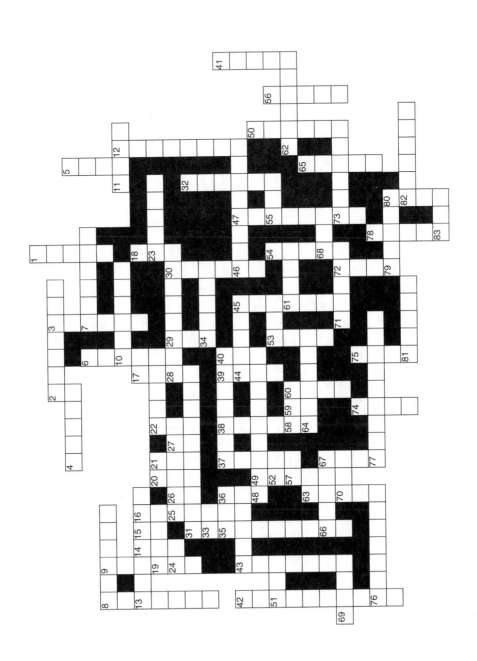

7. ROOT MULTIPLE CHOICE EXERCISE

Select the correct answer(s) and write the letter(s) of your choice in the space.

_____   1   The root for fat is
       (a)   lipo.
       (b)   litho.
       (c)   neuro.
       (d)   all of the above
       (e)   none of the above

_____   2.   The rectum is called
       (a)   behind.
       (b)   procto.
       (c)   ano.
       (d)   colo.
       (e)   entero.

_____   3.   Mast means
       (a)   muscle.
       (b)   chest.
       (c)   breast.
       (d)   all of the above
       (e)   none of the above

_____   4.   The root for ear is
       (a)   otic.
       (b)   optic.
       (c)   oto.
       (d)   ophthal.
       (e)   os.

_____   5.   The root for tube is
       (a)   naso.
       (b)   vaso.
       (c)   salpingo.
       (d)   oophoro.
       (e)   none of the above

_____   6. The root for head is
      (a) psyche.
      (b) cephalo.
      (c) cranio.
      (d) encephalo.
      (e) myelo.

_____   7. The root for joint is
      (a) osteo.
      (b) arthro.
      (c) rheumato.
      (d) all of the above
      (e) none of the above

_____   8. The root for abdomen is
      (a) laparo.
      (b) hystero.
      (c) litho.
      (d) all of the above
      (e) none of the above

_____   9. The word for pertaining to the kidney is
      (a) renal.
      (b) nephro.
      (c) pyelo.
      (d) all of the above
      (e) none of the above

_____   10. Vas is the root for
      (a) sac.
      (b) vein.
      (c) duct.
      (d) blood.
      (e) vessel.

_____   11. Choledocho means
      (a) bile duct or tube.
      (b) liver duct or tube.
      (c) egg duct or tube.
      (d) lung duct or tube.
      (e) none of the above

_____ 12.   Uretero refers to
(a)   joint.
(b)   artery.
(c)   urethra.
(d)   uterus.
(e)   ureter.

_____ 13.   The root oste means
(a)   mouth.
(b)   straight.
(c)   bone.
(d)   all of the above
(e)   none of the above

_____ 14.   Another word for uterus is
(a)   hystero.
(b)   womb.
(c)   metro.
(d)   all of the above
(e)   none of the above

_____ 15.   The large intestine is called
(a)   laparo.
(b)   sigmoid.
(c)   colo.
(d)   all of the above
(e)   none of the above

_____ 16.   Colpo is the root for
(a)   colon.
(b)   vagina.
(c)   rib.
(d)   all of the above
(e)   none of the above

_____ 17.   The root for heart is
(a)   cardio.
(b)   costo.
(c)   chondro.
(d)   all of the above
(e)   none of the above

_____   18.   Myo means
        (a)   bone marrow.
        (b)   muscle.
        (c)   spinal cord.
        (d)   eardrum.
        (e)   measure.

_____   19.   The root(s) for the large pelvic bone is/are
        (a)   illeo.
        (b)   ilio.
        (c)   ileo.
        (d)   all of the above
        (e)   none of the above

_____   20.   Prostato means
        (a)   vein.
        (b)   prostate.
        (c)   prostrate.
        (d)   all of the above
        (e)   none of the above

_____   21.   The root broncho means
        (a)   stomach.
        (b)   mouth.
        (c)   abdomen.
        (d)   all of the above
        (e)   none of the above

_____   22.   The root orchi means
        (a)   prostate.
        (b)   testicles.
        (c)   ovary.
        (d)   all of the above
        (e)   none of the above

_____   23.   The oviduct is also called
        (a)   fallopian tube.
        (b)   salpingo.
        (c)   egg tube.
        (d)   all of the above
        (e)   none of the above

_____ 24. The root for a portion of the small intestine is
  (a) illeo.
  (b) ilio.
  (c) ileo.
  (d) all of the above
  (e) none of the above

_____ 25. The root for eye is
  (a) otic.
  (b) oto.
  (c) ophthalmo.
  (d) all of the above
  (e) none of the above

_____ 26. The root derma means
  (a) outer.
  (b) hard.
  (c) skin.
  (d) all of the above
  (e) none of the above

_____ 27. The root(s) for man is/are
  (a) anoid.
  (b) arthro.
  (c) android.
  (d) all of the above
  (e) none of the above

_____ 28. The root myelo means
  (a) bone marrow.
  (b) muscle.
  (c) spinal cord.
  (d) all of the above
  (e) none of the above

_____ 29. The root ano means
  (a) appendix.
  (b) rectum.
  (c) anus.
  (d) all of the above
  (e) none of the above

30. The root(s) for nerve is/are
    (a) necro.
    (b) nephro.
    (c) noxi.
    (d) all of the above
    (e) none of the above

31. The root(s) for artery is/are
    (a) arterio.
    (b) arthro.
    (c) phlebo.
    (d) all of the above
    (e) none of the above

32. The root gynec means
    (a) woman.
    (b) female.
    (c) feminine.
    (d) all of the above
    (e) none of the above

33. The root(s) for nose is/are
    (a) scento.
    (b) rhino.
    (c) naso.
    (d) all of the above
    (e) none of the above

34. The root(s) for stomach is/are
    (a) laparo.
    (b) gastro.
    (c) colo.
    (d) all of the above
    (e) none of the above

35. The root chondro means
    (a) the colon.
    (b) muscle.
    (c) cartilage.
    (d) all of the above
    (e) none of the above

_____ 36. Which of the following pertain to the root for kidney?

(a) ren

(b) nephro

(c) renal

(d) all of the above

(e) none of the above

_____ 37. The root cranio means

(a) freeze.

(b) skull.

(c) head.

(d) all of the above

(e) none of the above

_____ 38. The root cholecysto means

(a) gall duct.

(b) gall vessel.

(c) gallbladder.

(d) all of the above

(e) none of the above

_____ 39. The root for the small intestine is

(a) gastro.

(b) entero.

(c) colo.

(d) procto.

(e) none of the above

_____ 40. The root andro means

(a) joint.

(b) artery.

(c) man.

(d) all of the above

(e) none of the above

_____ 41. The heart is located in the

(a) abdominal cavity.

(b) cranial cavity.

(c) chest cavity.

(d) all of the above

(e) none of the above

_____   42.   The root hepato means
     (a)   bone marrow.
     (b)   muscle.
     (c)   uterus.
     (d)   all of the above
     (e)   none of the above

_____   43.   The root stomato means
     (a)   stomach.
     (b)   mouth.
     (c)   abdomen.
     (d)   all of the above
     (e)   none of the above

_____   44.   The root cysto means
     (a)   bladder.
     (b)   rib.
     (c)   cartilage.
     (d)   all of the above
     (e)   none of the above

_____   45.   The coccyx is located in/on the
     (a)   abdomen.
     (b)   spine.
     (c)   head.
     (d)   body trunk.
     (e)   none of the above

_____   46.   The root for rib is
     (a)   costo.
     (b)   cardio.
     (c)   chondro.
     (d)   all of the above
     (e)   none of the above

_____   47.   The root thyro means
     (a)   trachea.
     (b)   chest.
     (c)   thyroid.
     (d)   all of the above
     (e)   none of the above

_____ 48.   The root for bile duct is
        (a)   choledocho.
        (b)   cholecysto.
        (c)   cholesalpingo.
        (d)   all of the above
        (e)   none of the above

_____ 49.   The root procto means
        (a)   prostate.
        (b)   kidney pelvis.
        (c)   rectum.
        (d)   all of the above
        (e)   none of the above

_____ 50.   The root broncho means
        (a)   bronchus.
        (b)   a wild horse.
        (c)   bladder.
        (d)   all of the above
        (e)   none of the above

8. ROOT IDENTIFICATION EXERCISE

Write the proper root for the following words.

1. bile _____

2. cancer _____

3. color _____

4. menses _____

5. eardrum or tympanic membrane _____

6. mouth _____

7. ovary _____

8. cornea _____

9. fungus _____

10. nail or claw _____

11. pharynx_____

12. rib _____

13. pleura or side _____

14. column of vertebrae in spine _____

15. walk_____

16. eyelid_____

17. tailbone _____

18. lung_____

19. connective tissue _____

20. cell _____

21. head _____

22. brain _____

23. joint _____

24. mucus _____

25. blood_____

26. cartilage_____

27. heart _____

28. skin _____

29. stone _____

30. tongue _____

31. tooth _____

32. vagina _____

33. blood vessel _____

34. bone _____

35. clot _____

36. child _____

37. ear _____

38. eye _____

39. foot _____

40. fungus _____

41. kidney _____

42. mind _____

43. nerve _____

44. ovary _____

45. pelvis of kidney _____

46. pertaining to the kidney _____

47. tube _____

48. vessel, duct _____

49. fat _____

50. uterus _____

THE MALE INTERNAL ORGAN EXERCISE

Identify the parts shown by the line to them.

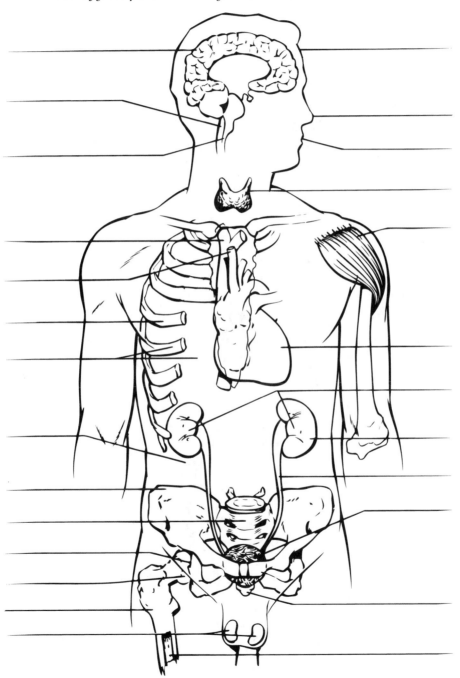

THE FEMALE INTERNAL ORGAN EXERCISE

Identify the parts shown by the line to them.

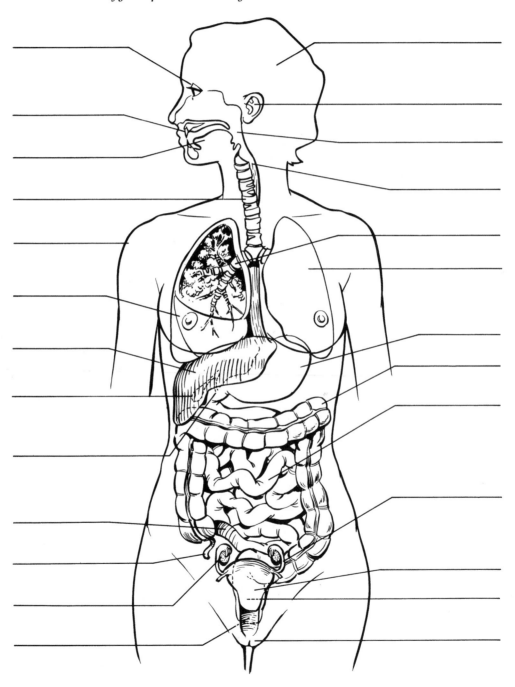

PUTTING IT ALL
TOGETHER

6

At this point, you are ready to use all of the prefixes, suffixes, and roots or stems you learned in the previous chapters. This chapter consists of a variety of exercises using all of these elements, as well as the locations, positions, and anatomy covered. You will also "create" words, using word elements you know.

Now is the time for you to use a medical dictionary, because some new terms are combined with the "old" in this chapter. It may be helpful to place a checkmark beside a word in the dictionary the first time you look it up, whether to verify the spelling or definition. If you look it up again, you will find your checkmark and know it has not "stuck" in your mind. If that is the case, highlight it. Finding a highlighted word indicates it is used often and is difficult to learn or remember. Write it correctly on an alpha-blocked list at your desk; when you no longer need to check the spelling, delete it from that list. This hint will save time and will also enforce the word in your mind.

When you run across a word element you are unfamiliar with, you should be able to make an educated guess as to where it is located, what system it is in, what specialty it applies to, or if it is a surgical or diagnostic term by using the terms you know and putting the new one in context with the old.

At the completion of this chapter, you will be able to read, pronounce, and understand a wide variety of medical reports, papers, and dictation. You will also be able to use a medical dictionary for checking your spelling, and you will find your spelling, as well as your vocabulary, constantly improving.

1. REVIEW DEFINITION EXERCISE

Define each component and then define the entire word.

1. post _____ partum _____

   postpartum _____.

2. dys _____ peps _____ ia _____

   dyspepsia _____.

3. audio _____ meter _____

   audiometer _____.

4. pneumo _____ centesis_____

   pneumocentesis _____.

5. a _____ phas _____ia_____

   aphasia _____.

6. procto _____ ptosis _____

   proctoptosis _____.

7. arthro _____ desis_____

   arthrodesis _____.

8. hernio _____ rrhaphy_____

   herniorrhaphy _____.

9. micro _____ scope_____

   microscope _____.

10. oophor _____ ectomy_____

    oophorectomy _____.

11. metro _____ rrhag _____ ia _____

metrorrhagia _____.

12. crypt _____orchi(d) _____ ism_____

cryptorchidism _____.

13. dipl_____ opia _____

diplopia _____.

14. necr _____ opsy _____

necropsy _____.

15. hyper _____ trophy _____

hypertrophy _____.

16. sub _____ cutane _____ ous _____

subcutaneous _____.

17. endo _____ card _____ium _____

endocardium _____.

18. trans _____ mit _____

transmit _____.

19. hyster _____ ectomy_____

hysterectomy _____.

20. lumbo _____ sacr_____ al_____

lumbosacral _____.

21. hepat _____ itis_____

hepatitis _____.

22. quadri _____ pleg _____ ia _____

    quadriplegia _____.

23. gastro _____ scope _____

    gastroscope _____.

24. macro _____ gloss_____ ia _____

    macroglossia _____.

25. dent _____ algia_____

    dentalgia _____.

2. REVIEW DEFINITION EXERCISE

Define each component and then define the entire word.

1. peri _____ metr _____ ium_____

   perimetrium _____.

2. epi _____ cyst _____ itis _____

   epicystitis _____.

3. micro _____ card _____ ia _____

   microcardia _____

4. dys _____ pnea _____.

   dyspnea _____.

5. hypo_____ therm_____ia_____.

   hypothermia _____.

6. auto_____ bio_____ graph_____

    ic   _____ al_____.

    autobiographical   _____.

7. leuco _____ derma _____

    leucoderma   _____.

8. hyper _____ alg _____ ic_____

    hyperalgic _____.

9. neuro _____ genic_____

    neurogenic _____.

10. histo _____ path _____ology _____

    histopathology_____.

11. thorac   _____ ostomy _____

    thoracostomy _____.

12. hemat _____ oma _____

    hematoma _____.

13. psycho _____ path_____ ic _____

    psychopathic _____.

14. gastro _____ scopy_____

    gastroscopy _____.

15. blephar_____ ectomy_____

    blepharectomy _____.

16. chole _____ cysto _____ gram _____

     cholecystogram _____.

17. hypo _____ esthesia _____

     hypoesthesia _____.

18. nephr _____ otomy _____

     nephrotomy _____.

19. pharyng _____ itis _____

     pharyngitis _____.

20. cysto _____ lith _____ osis _____

     cystolithosis _____.

21. cyst _____ ectomy _____

     cystectomy _____.

22. myo _____ oma _____

     myoma _____.

23. osteo _____ scler _____osis _____

     osteosclerosis _____.

24. arthr _____ ectomy _____

     arthrectomy _____.

25. noct _____ ambul _____ ism _____

     noctambulism _____.

3. REVIEW DEFINITION EXERCISE

Define each component and then define the entire word.

1. psycho _____ genic _____

    psychogenic _____.

2   hemi _____ nephro _____ectomy _____

    heminephrectomy _____.

3. necro _____ phobia _____

    necrophobia _____.

4. angio _____ card _____ itis _____

    angiocarditis _____.

5. tachy _____ card _____ ia _____

    tachycardia _____.

6. cyan _____ osis _____

    cyanosis _____.

7. melan _____ oma _____

    melanoma _____.

8. hemo _____ ptysis _____

    hemoptysis _____.

9. dys _____ meno _____ rrhea _____

    dysmenorrhea_____.

10. osteo _____ arthro_____ itis _____

osteoarthritis _____.

11. hemo _____ pneumo _____ thorax_____

hemopneumothorax _____.

12. cardi _____ peri _____ pexy_____

cardiopericardiopexy _____.

13. salpingo _____ ectomy_____

salpingectomy_____.

14. intra _____ cost_____ al _____

intracostal _____.

15. osteo_____ myelo_____ itis _____

osteomyelitis _____.

16. masto _____ pexy_____

mastopexy _____.

17. sub _____ costal _____

subcostal_____.

18. poly _____ uria _____

polyuria _____.

19. pneumo _____ itis _____

pneumonitis _____.

20. chole _____ lith_____ osis_____

cholelithosis _____.

21. micro _____ hemat _____ uria _____

    microhematuria _____.

22. pyo _____ gen _____ ic _____

    pyogenic _____ . _____.

23. sub _____ lingu _____ al _____

    sublingual _____.

24. gluco _____ gen _____ ic _____

    glucogenic _____.

25. mono _____ neuro _____ al_____

    mononeural _____.

4. REVIEW DEFINITION EXERCISE

Define each component and then define the entire word.

1. phago _____ cyt _____ osis_____

   phagocytosis _____.

2. lipo _____ derm _____ ia _____

   lipodermia _____.

3. path _____ ology _____

   pathology _____.

4. taxi _____ derm_____

   taxidermy _____.

5. olig _____ uria _____

   oliguria _____.

6. oto _____ scope _____

   otoscope _____.

7. spire _____ meter _____

   spirometer _____.

8. neo _____ nat _____ al_____

   neonatal _____.

9. anti _____ pyre _____ tic _____

   antipyretic _____.

10. ante _____ partum_____

    antepartum _____.

11. ex _____ cise _____

    excise _____.

12. ovi _____ duct_____

    oviduct _____.

13. hypo _____ glyc _____ emia _____

    hypoglycemia _____.

14. hystero _____ pexy_____

    hysteropexy _____.

15. thrombo _____ cyto _____ penia_____

    thrombocytopenia _____

16. laparo _____ scope _____

    laparoscope   _____.

17. myc _____ ology _____

    mycology   _____.

18. anti _____ histo _____ gen_____ ic _____

    antihistogenic _____.

19. neuro _____ path_____ ic _____

    neuropathic   _____.

20. bilateral _____ crypt_____

    orchid _____ ectomy_____

    bilateral cryptorchidectomy _____.

21. nephro _____ lith_____ iasis _____

    nephrolithiasis   _____.

22. thrombo _____ phlebo _____ itis _____

    thrombophlebitis   _____.

23. phlebo _____ otomy _____

    phlebotomy   _____.

24. vas _____ ectomy _____

    vasectomy   _____.

25. pneumo _____ itis _____

    pneumonitis   _____.

5. *PUTTING IT ALL TOGETHER PUZZLE*

ACROSS

2. Difficult breathing
4. Double vision
6. Within the ribs
8. After birth
11. Surgical removal of an ovary
13. Condition of a dry mouth
15. Hidden or undescended testicle
17. Surgical removal of a joint
18. Instrument to check escape of (keeping it in place) blood
19. Above the kidney
20. Nourishment
22. Condition of a slow heart

DOWN

1. Inflammation of a joint
2. Condition of difficult or painful digestion
3. Incision or cutting of a vein
5. Fallen rectum
7. Scanty urine
8. Puncture of and removal of fluid from the lung
9. Bursting forth from the uterus—excessive uterine bleeding
10. Autopsy for animals
12. Blood making
14. Between the ribs
16. Condition of eating by or destruction of cells
21. Condition of absence or lack of speech

PUTTING IT ALL TOGETHER PUZZLE

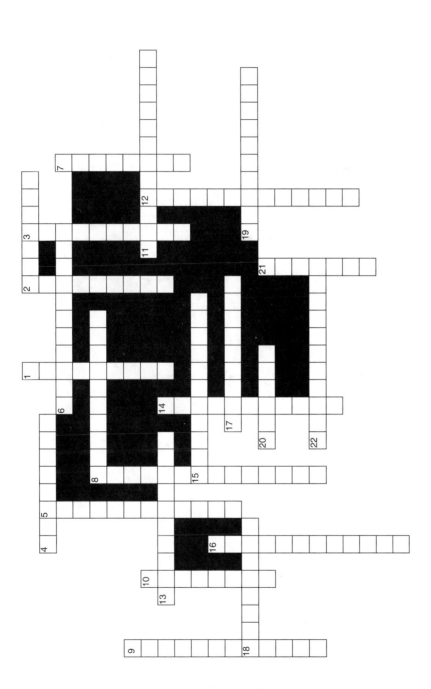

6. REVIEW COMPLETION EXERCISE

Fill in the blanks with the proper medical or surgical specialty(ies).

1.   Surgery on children   _____.

2.   Surgery on the heart _____.

3.   Surgery on the nervous system _____.

4.   Surgery on diseases of the mouth _____.

5.   Surgery on the skeletal system _____.

6.   Surgery on urinary tract_____.

7.   Treatment of the female reproductive system _____.

8.   Treatment of the mind   _____.

9.   Treatment of the aged _____.

10.   Treatment of cancers/malignancies_____.

11.   Treatment for asthma_____.

12.   Treatment for a heart attack _____.

13.   Sleep for surgery _____.

14.   Treatment of the eyes_____.

15.   Treatment of a blood disease _____.

16.   Treatment of the stomach/intestines _____.

17.   Treatment of diseases of the rectum _____.

18.   Treatment of overall health _____.

19.   Treatment of the skin _____ .

20.   Treatment of infertility in men _____ .

21.   Counseling for inherited diseases _____ .

22.   Treatment of hormonal problems _____ .

23.   Treatment of pregnancy/delivery _____ .

24.   X-rays _____ .

25.   Filling of a prescription _____ .

Fill in the blank with the word(s) that most correctly complete the sentence.

26.   Posterior means the same as _____ .

27.   A disease or infection of the blood is_____ .

28.   Inflammation of the heart from within is _____ .

29.   Angionecrosis is _____ .

30.   A very fast heart is _____ .

31.   Meningitis is _____ .

32.   The outer layer of skin is called the _____ .

33.   Inflamed skin is _____ .

34.   A condition of blood in the oviduct is _____ .

35.   The surgical removal of the gallbladder is_____ .

36.   Water/fluid in a hernia or sac is a _____ .

37.   A ruptured uterus is _____ .

38.   Hormones are secreted by which system? _____.

39.   Water on the brain is _____.

40.   Rachicentesis means _____.

41.   A sleep seizure, or an uncontrollable desire to sleep, is called ____

_____.

42.   A condition of nail eating (or biting) is _____.

43.   An abnormal fear of heights is _____.

44.   The study of the inside of the brain is _____.

45.   Upon the skin is _____.

46.   Pertaining to behind the sternum, or breastbone, is _____.

47.   To be partly, or about half, away is to be _____.

48.   Of a thin skin is _____.

49.   If you are supine, you are _____.

50.   Pertaining to the back of the body is _____.

Define and explain each procedure listed.

51.   colostomy closure _____.

52.   tubal anastomosis-laparoscopy _____.

_____.

53.   exploratory laparotomy _____

_____.

54. tympanomastoidectomy _____

_____.

55. microsuspension laryngoscopy _____

_____.

56. adenoidectomy _____.

57. cystoscopy _____.

58. right retrograde pyelogram _____.

59. excision peritoneal lesions _____.

60. palatoplasty_____.

61. parotidectomy_____.

62. colecystectomy _____.

63. subtemporal/suboccipital craniotomy resection _____.

64. arthroscopy_____.

65. costoscopy, bilateral and retrograde _____.

66. blepharoplasty _____.

67. cholecystectomy_____.

68. bilateral mastectomy _____.

69. tonsillectomy _____.

70. urethrolithotomy _____.

7. REVIEW OF PARAGRAPHS—TRANSLATING FROM MEDICAL TO LAY TERMS

Read each paragraph. Define the italicized words, and then paraphrase the answer in lay terms, using the medical word definitions to explain.

1. *Diagnostic* impression: Extensive *diverticulosis* and focal *diverticulitis*, with intramural abscess formation, was found in the sigmoid colon.

   diagnostic _____.

   diverticulosis _____.

   diverticulitis _____.

   _____

   _____

   _____

   _____.

2. Surgery: Exploratory *laparotomy*, colon *resection*.

   laparotomy _____.

   resection _____.

   _____

   _____

   _____

   _____.

3. Under general *anesthesia,* the patient was prepped and draped. The abdomen was entered through a *lower midline* incision.

    anesthesia_____.

    lower midline   _____.

    _____

    _____

    _____.

4. Spleen was grossly normal to *palpation.* There was *inflammation* about the sigmoid colon and it was *adherent* to the *lateral pelvic* wall.

    palpation _____.

    inflammation   _____.

    adherent   _____.

    lateral   _____.

    pelvic   _____.

    _____

    _____

    _____

    _____.

5. An elliptical incision was used to perform a modified *radical mastectomy*. *Dissection* was carried out *medially* through the *sternal* borders, *superiorly* to the *infraclavicular* area, *laterally* to the latissimus dorsi and *inferiorly* to the insertion of the rectus muscle... two catheters were left in the *subcutaneous* area and brought out through the skin and ligated with *2-0* silk ties.(*Note:* 2-0 is pronounced two-ought.)

radical _____.

mastectomy_____.

dissection _____.

medially _____.

sternal _____.

superiorly _____.

infraclavicular_____.

laterally _____.

inferiorly _____.

subcutaneous _____.

2-0 _____.

_____

_____

_____

_____

_____

_____.

6. Twenty *axillary* lymph node sections from all four *quadrants* are examined and are negative for *metastatic carcinoma*. They show only benign *histiocytosis* and *hyperplasia*. Pathological examination of the sections revealed *interlobular sclerosis, duct ectasia,* focal adenosis, and *sclerosing adenosis.*

axillary _____.

quadrants _____.

metastatic _____.

carcinoma _____.

histiocytosis_____.

hyperplasia _____.

interlobular_____.

sclerosis _____.

duct _____.

ectasia _____.

sclerosing adenosis _____.

_____

_____

_____

_____

_____.

8. REVIEW OF PARAGRAPHS—TRANSLATING FROM LAY TO MEDICAL TERMS

Read each paragraph. Write the proper medical word in for the lay term, using words you already know. You may "create a word." Then write a short summary using the medical words of the lay description above.

1. The victim had cold, blue skin, a very rapid heart rate, and pain in the body.

Cold, blue skin   _____ .

Very rapid heart rate   _____ .

Pain in the body _____ .

_____

_____

_____ .

2. Symptoms included overactivity (new word—*hyperkinesis*) or agitation, excessive thirst, vomited or coughed up blood, and blood in the urine.

Overactivity_____ .

Excessive thirst   _____ .

Vomiting blood   _____ .

Blood in the urine   _____ .

_____

_____

_____

_____ .

3. After a head injury, the patient had a rapid flow of blood from the nose and throat, a loss of feeling, paralysis of one side of the body, a slow heart rate, and was vomiting blood.

Rapid flow of blood _____.

Nose and throat _____.

Loss of feeling_____.

Paralysis of one side of the body _____.

Slow heart rate _____.

Vomiting blood _____.

_____

_____

_____

_____.

4. The nosebleed came from high blood pressure and failure of the blood to clot.

Nosebleed (new word—*epistaxis,* literally a dropping upon) ____

_____.

High blood pressure _____.

Failure of the blood to clot _____.

_____

_____

_____.

POSTTEST

Match the best lettered definition with the numbered word.

_____	1.	antero	a.	pus
_____	2.	hetero	b.	under, low
_____	3.	hypo	c.	in front
_____	4.	intra	d.	death
_____	5.	lepto	e.	before
_____	6.	medio	f.	bone
_____	7.	mega	g.	exceptionally large
_____	8.	angio	h.	sleep
_____	9.	narc	i.	between
_____	10.	necro	j.	thin
_____	11.	laparo	k.	from, away
_____	12.	abs	l.	fast
_____	13.	ortho	m.	different
_____	14.	pan	n.	man
_____	15.	pyo	o.	within
_____	16.	semi	p.	vessel
_____	17.	ad	q.	over, high
_____	18.	tachy	r.	freeze, cold
_____	19.	hyper	s.	partly, about half

_____	20.	vari	t.	straight
_____	21.	inter	u.	middle
_____	22.	brady	v.	slow
_____	23.	cryo	w.	near, toward
_____	24.	ante	x.	all
_____	25.	andro	y.	loins, abdomen
_____	26.	osteo	z.	different

Fill in the blanks.

27.   Adenopathy is a disease of a _____.

28. 29.   A lipochilectomy is the _____ of a fat _____.

30.   A cholecystectomy is the surgical removal of the _____.

31. 32.   Hematuria is _____ in the _____.

33. 34.   Histology is the _____ of _____.

35. 36.   Keratosis is a _____ of the_____.

37.   An instrument to examine the abdomen is called a _____

_____.

38.   Under the tongue is _____.

39–41.   Osteoarthritis is _____ of the _____ and

_____.

42.   The word meaning pertaining to the ear is _____.

Fill in the blanks.

43. 44.   Thrombosis is a _____ of _____.

45.   Psychogenic means _____ by the mind.

46. 47.   Rhinorrhea is a _____ from the _____.

48. 49.   Tinea pedis is _____ of the _____.

50. 51.   Afebrile means _____.

Fill in the blanks with the name of the proper medical or surgical specialist.

52.   Surgery on the nervous system_____

53.   Surgery on diseases of the mouth _____

54.   Treatment of the female reproductive system_____

55.   Treatment of the aged _____

56.   Treatment of cancers and malignancies_____

57.   Treatment of a blood disease_____

58.   Treatment of the stomach/intestines_____

59.   Treatment of diseases of the rectum_____

60.   Treatment of infertility in men _____

61.   Counseling for inherited diseases_____

62.   Treatment of hormonal problems _____

Match the best lettered definition with the numbered word.

_____	63.	amphi	a.	tooth
_____	64.	cuti	b.	tongue
_____	65.	cephalo	c.	right
_____	66.	linguo	d.	white
_____	67.	pyelo	e.	difficult, painful
_____	68.	dextro	f.	red
_____	69.	thrombo	g.	cause
_____	70.	erythro	h.	about, both sides
_____	71.	myco	i.	outside, away
_____	72.	cilia	j.	fungus
_____	73.	ora	k.	opening/mouth
_____	74.	etio	l.	clot
_____	75.	alb	m.	fungus
_____	76.	tinea	n.	head
_____	77.	ambi	o.	lip
_____	78.	dys	p.	small hair, eyelash
_____	79.	chilo	q.	blood vessel, vessel, duct
_____	80.	ex	r.	both
_____	81.	dent	s.	renal pelvis
_____	82.	vaso	t.	skin

Multiple choice: Select the best answer(s).

_____ 83. Choledocho means _____ duct or tube.
- (a) bile
- (b) liver
- (c) egg
- (d) all of above
- (e) none of above

_____ 84. Ureto refers to
- (a) joint.
- (b) artery.
- (c) man.
- (d) all of above
- (e) none of above

_____ 85. The word metro also means
  (a) womb.
  (b) hystero.
  (c) uterus.
  (d) all of above
  (e) none of above

_____ 86. The large intestine is called
  (a) laparo.
  (b) gastro.
  (c) colo.
  (d) all of above
  (e) none of above

_____ 87. Colpo is
  (a) colon.
  (b) vagina.
  (c) rib.
  (d) all of above
  (e) none of above

_____ 88. Myo means
  (a) bone marrow.
  (b) muscle.
  (c) spinal cord.
  (d) all of above
  (e) none of above

_____ 89. The large pelvic bone is called
  (a) illeo.
  (b) ilio.
  (c) ileo.
  (d) all of above
  (e) none of above

_____ 90. Broncho means
  (a) stomach.
  (b) mouth.
  (c) abdomen.
  (d) all of above
  (e) none of above

_____   91.   Orchi means

    (a)   prostate.

    (b)   testicles.

    (c)   ovary.

    (d)   all of above

    (e)   none of above

_____   92.   The oviduct is also called

    (a)   fallopian tube

    (b)   salpingo

    (c)   egg passage/tube

    (d)   all of above

    (e)   none of above

_____   93.   The word for intestine is

    (a)   illeo.

    (b)   ilio.

    (c)   entero.

    (d)   all of above

    (e)   none of above

_____   94.   The word for eye is

    (a)   otic.

    (b)   oto.

    (c)   ophthalmo.

    (d)   all of above

    (e)   none of above

_____   95.   Myelo means

    (a)   bone marrow.

    (b)   muscle.

    (c)   spinal cord.

    (d)   all of above

    (e)   none of above

_____   96.   Ano means

    (a)   appendix.

    (b)   man.

    (c)   anus.

    (d)   all of above

    (e)   none of above

_____ 97. The word for nerve is

       (a)   neuro.

       (b)   naso.

       (c)   nevoid.

       (d)   all of above

       (e)   none of above

_____ 98. The word for artery is

       (a)   arterio.

       (b)   arthro.

       (c)   phlebo.

       (d)   all of above

       (e)   none of above

_____ 99. Which of the following refer to the kidney?

       (a)   ren.

       (b)   nephro.

       (c)   renal.

       (d)   all of above

       (e)   none of above

_____ 100. Cranio means

       (a)   encephalo.

       (b)   skull.

       (c)   cephalo.

       (d)   all of above

       (e)   none of above

GLOSSARY

These are all the word pieces used in the book—prefixes, suffixes, and roots/stems—and their definitions. Positions and locations are also listed. There are no words as such, like cardiology, amniocentesis, etc. They are in the index.

a   without, from, away
ab   from, away
abs   from, away
ace(a, o)   cure
acro   top, extremity, height
ad   near to, near, toward
aden(o)   gland
aero   air, gas
al   of, pertaining to
alb   white
algia   process, condition, presence of pain
ambi   both
ambul   walk
amphi   about, both, on both sides
an   without
andr(o)   man
angi(o)   vessel
ano   anus

ante   before
anterior   pertaining to front or in front of body/body part
anter(o)   in front, the front
anti   against
append   appendix, outgrowth
archy   rule
arter(i, io)   artery
arthr(o)   joint
ate   to become
atric(s)   cure
auto   self

bi   two, double, both
bilateral   of, pertaining to both (2) sides
bio   life
blephar(o)   eyelid/eyelash
brady   slow
bronch(o)   bronchus
brun   brown

carcin(o)   cancer
card(i, io)   heart
caudal   of or pertaining to lower part of spinal column
cavity   any hollow space
cele   swelling, hernia, protrusion
centesis   act/process of puncture of and withdrawal of fluid
cephal(o)   head
cephalad   toward, near, near to the head
chil(o)   lip
chlor(o)   green
chol(e, a, o)   bile, gall
cholecyst(o)   gallbladder
choledoch(o)   gall, bile duct
chondr(o)   cartilage
chro   color
cide   kill
cili   small hair, eyelash/lid
cilia   process, condition, presence of small hair, eyelash/lid
cili(o)   small hair, eyelash/lid
cirrh(o)   orange
cise   cut

cle   small

col(o)   colon

colp(o)   vagina

colpos   vagina (mouth)

corp(o)   body

corpus   body

cost(o)   rib

cranial   of or pertaining to skull

crani(o)   skull

cry(o)   freeze, cold

crypt   hidden

cule   small

cut   skin

cuti   skin

cutane   skin

cyano   blue

cyst(o)   sac, bladder

cyt(o)   cell

cyte   cell

de   from, remove

dent(o)(i)   tooth

dont   tooth

derm(a)   skin

desis   act/process of binding

dextr(o)   right

di   two, double, both

dia   across, through, between, completely

dipl(o)   two, double

distal   of or pertaining to farthest from point of attachment

doch(o)   duct, tube, to lead

dolicho   long

dorsal   of or pertaining to the back of body/body part

dorsal lithotomy position   on back, knees raised well over buttocks, arms
    crossed over chest, feet in stirrups, flexed and rotated outward

dorsal position   lying on back, legs straight, head in line with body,
    arms alongside body, palms down

dorsal recumbent position   lying on back, head in line with body, knees
    bent 45° angle, arms alongside body, palms down

duct   to lead, tube

du(o)   two, double

dyne   pain
dynia   of process, condition, presence of pain
dys   difficult, painful

ec   on the outside, external
ect(o)   on the outside, external
ecta   extension, dilation
ectasis   act/process of extension, or dilation
ectomy   surgical removal of
ectop(y)   displacement, malposition, especially congenital
ectopic   of being out of place
emesis   act/process of vomiting
emia   process, condition, presence of condition of the blood
encephal(o)   of or pertaining to brain
end(o)   inner, inside within, inward
ens   of, belonging to
enter(o)   intestine
epi   upon, among
eryth(r, ro)   red
es(o)   inward, within
esophag(o)   esophagus (within/swallow, eat)
esthesia   process, condition, presence of sensation, feeling
eti(o)   cause
eu   good, well, normal
eum   a place where
ex(o)   outside, out, away
external   of or pertaining to outside
extra   outside of

febr   fever, fire
fibr   connective tissue
fibr(o)   connective tissue
form   resembling, shaped
Fowler position   head up, knees at 45° angle, legs down
ful   full of

gastr(o)   stomach
gen(e)   produce, cause
genic   of a cause/production, causing, producing, caused, produced
ger(io, at, ont, onto)   old age
glob(o)   ball, globe

gloss(o)   tongue
gluc(o)   sweet, sugar
glyc(o)   sweet, sugar
gram   instrument that records lines, drawings, makes a record
graph   lines, drawings, writing, a recording, or a record
gyn(o)   woman
gyne   woman
gynec(o)   woman

hem(o)   blood
hemat(o)   blood
hemi   half (usually lateral; 1 side)
hepat(o)   liver
herni(o)   hernia, a rupture
heter(o)   different
hex(a)   six
hist(o)   tissue
hydr(o)   water, water-like fluid
hyper   too much, over, high
hypo   too little, under, low
hyster(o)   uterus

ia   process, condition, presence of
iasis   act/ process, condition, presence of
ic   of
icle   little
id   condition of (morbid)
ileo   ileum (part of small intestine)
ilio   ilium (large pelvic bone)
inferior   below
infra   below, beneath
ino   within
inter   between
internal   of or pertaining to inside
intra   within
ipsi   same, self
ism   process of
ist   one who
itis   inflammation of, infection
ium   small
ize   away, remove, free from, cleanse

kerat(o)   horn, cornea

kine   movement

knee-chest position   chest and side of face down on table, buttocks elevated, knees completely flexed with top of feet on table

lapar(o)   loins, abdomen

lateral   of or pertaining to side of body/body part

lateral position   lying on either side, with body at edge of table, lower leg slightly flexed (depending on side lying on), upper leg straight, if a pillow is placed between legs, or fully flexed for comfort and ease of examination, arms outstretched at right angles for support

later(o)   to the side of

lepsy   seizure

lept(o)   thin

leuc(o)   white

leuk(o)   white

lev(o)   left

lingu(o)   tongue

lip(o)   fat

lith(o)   stone

logy   study of, science

lute   yellow (corpus luteum, like an egg yolk)

lyse   wash, rinse

lysis   act/process of destruction, decomposition, dissolution; gradual abatement or receding or lessening of disease symptoms; of washing, rinsing (lyse)

lytic   belonging to, of, pertaining to dissolution, destruction, gradual abatement, or lessening of the symptoms of disease

macr(o)   excessively large or long

mal   bad

malacia   process, presence, or condition of morbid softening of part or morbid craving for highly spiced foods

mast(o)   breast

medial   of or pertaining to medio (middle), toward the midline, or middle of body or any body part

med(i, io)   middle

mega   large (exceptionally)

megaly   enlargement—abnormal, exceptional

melan   black

meninges   membranes over brain and spinal cord

men(o)   menses, menstruation

mes(o)   middle
meter   to measure
metr(o)   uterus
metry   measurement
micr(o)   small
midline   imaginary line dividing body/body part into right and left sides
   through the center
mit   sent/send
mon(o)   one, single
morbid   of, affected with or causing disease, unhealthy, diseased,
   unwholesome
muc(o)   mucus
multi   many
my(o)   muscle
myc(o)   fungus
myelo   bone marrow, spinal cord
myo   muscle
myring(o)   tympanic membrane/eardrum

narc(o)   sleep
nas(o)   nose
necr(o)   death/dead
neo   new
nephr(o)   kidney
neur(o)   nerve
noct   night
nost   return home or to the familiar
nox(i)   injurious agent, act, influence
nox   night (rarely)

obstetri   midwife
ocul(o)   eye
oda   like, a resemblance, similar to
odes   like, a resemblance, similar to
oid   resembling, resembling form
ola   small
ole   small
olig(o)   few, scanty, small
ology   study of, science
oma   growth, tumor
onc(o, os)   mass, swelling, tumor
onychia   process, presence, condition of (finger/toenail)

onych(o)   nail (finger/toe)
oophor(o)   ovary
ophthalm(o)   eye
opisth(o)   backward, behind, located behind
optic   eye (belonging to or of)
ora   mouth, opening
ori   mouths, openings
orchi(o)   testicle, testis
oro   an opening or mouth
orth(o)   straight
os   opening, mouth, or mouth-like opening
osis   (morbid) process, condition, disease
oste(o)   bone
ostomy   mouth-like opening or incision formed for drainage
ot(i, o)   ear
otic   of, pertaining to ear
otomy   incision, cutting
ous   of, having
ov(a, i, um)   egg

pan   all
para   beside, near, beyond, apart from
parietal   of or pertaining to wall of a body structure
parous   giving birth to, bearing
partum   birth, delivery
path   disease, suffering
pathy   disease, suffering
ped (Greek)   child
ped (Latin)   foot, feet
pedia   process, presence, condition of child—education
penia   process, condition, presence of too few
pep(s)   digest, cook
peri   around
peripheral   of or pertaining to near the surface
pexy   surgical fixation
phag(o)   swallowing, eating
pharyng(o)   pharynx
phasia   of the process, condition, presence of speech
phleb(o)   vein
phobia   process, condition, presence of abnormal fear, dread
phoresis   act/process of or to carry, bear, transmission

phyll   leaf
plasm   anything formed
plast   anything formed
plasty   repair, molding, forming
pleur(o)   rib, side, pleura
pleura   membrane lining walls of chest cavity
pnea   breathing, breath
pneum(o)   lung, air
pod   foot, feet
poie   making
poly   many, much, excessive amount
post   after
posterior   back of body/body part
poster(o)   behind, the back of
pre   before
proct(o)   rectum
prone position   lying face down, opposite of supine
prostat(o)   prostate
proximal   of or pertaining to nearest point of attachment
pseud(o)   false
psyche, psych(o)   mind
ptosis   act/process of dropping of organ—abnormal placement of organ
ptysis   act/process of spitting, saliva
purpur   purple
pyel(o)   kidney/renal pelvis
pyo   pus
pyr(o)   fever, fire

quadr(o, u)   four, ¼ th

rachia   of spinal fluid
rachi   spine, column of vertebrae
ren(i)   kidney
renal   of or pertaining to the kidney
retr(o)   behind, located behind
rhin(o)   nose
rrhage   bursting forth
rrhagia   process, condition, presence of bursting forth
rrhaphy   suture, repair
rrhea   flow
rrhexis   act of a break, rupture

sacr(o)   sacrum
salping(o)   tube
schiz   split
scler(e, o)   hard, hardening
scope   instrument to examine
scopy   examine, observation, to examine
semi   partly, about or almost half
sep(i, t)   rotten, putrid, disease-causing organism(s) or bacteria
sex(i)   six
Sims position   lying on left side, knees bent toward abdomen
sis   act/process of
sophy   wisdom, art, skill
spasm   involuntary muscular act, convulsion, twitching, a tic
specul(o)   cave, hole
spire   breath/breathing
splen(o)   spleen
stalsis   act/process of constriction, or compression
static   standing, placed, pooled
stasis   act/process of standing, pooling, stagnation (refers to blood)
stat   standing, placed
stat (abbr.)   statim, at once
staxis   dropping, fall in drops
sten(o)   narrow
stern(o)   breast bone/sternum
stom, stoma   opening into, a mouth, artificial opening
stomat(o)   opening into, mouth, artificial opening
sub   under
sui   self
super   above, over
superior   above, over
supine position   lying on back, legs straight, head in line with body,
     arms alongside body, palms down
supine   lying on back
supra   above, over

tach(y, o)   fast
tax(o)   arrangement, arrange, order
taxi(s)   arrangement, arrange, order
tele   distance, far away, at a distance
tetra   four
therm   heat
thorac(o)   chest, thorax

thromb(o)   clot
thyr(o)   thyroid
tic   belonging to, of, pertaining to
tic   root for spasm
tinea   fungus
tomy   cutting, incision
topy   place
trache(o)   trachea
trans   across, through, beyond
Trendelenberg position   on back with knees flexed over lower break of
     examination table, arms alongside body, palms down, head and body
     higher than feet, or legs/feet elevated, body prone
tri   three, triple
trophy   nourishment
tropic   of turning toward, tending to turn or change
tropism   act of turning toward, tending to turn or change; growth
     response stimulus

ule   small
ulous   full of, characterized by
ulum(s)   small
uni   one, single
ur(e)   urine
ureter(o)   ureter
uria   of process, condition, presence in the urine
urticaria   process, condition, presence of hives
uter(o)   uterus, womb

vari   different
vas(o)   blood vessel /vessel/duct
ventral   of or pertaining to the front of the body/body part
visceral   of or pertaining to structures found inside the body

xanth(o)   yellow
xero   dry

INDEX

A/an, 1, 2, 26, 36, 37, 57, 99,152, 181
Ab, 57, 181
Abs, 5, 57, 181
Ace (a,o), 181
Acro, 14, 55, 181
Ad, 5, 55, 60, 181
Aden(o), 118
Aero, 25, 59, 181
Aerospace medicine, 25
Al, 3, 13, 14, 39, 60, 61, 63, 90, 181
Alb, 8, 58, 181
Algia, 90, 181
Allergist, 26, 30
Allergy, 26, 30, 31,
Ambi, 8, 55, 57, 181
Ambul, 199, 181
Ambulatory medicine, 28
Amphi, 8, 55, 181
An(o), 117, 121, 181
Ana, 19
Anatomy, 19,
Andr(o), 6, 59, 181
Anesthesiologist, 26
Anesthesiology, 26
Angi(o), 5, 118, 181
Ano, 117, 181

Ante, 6, 55, 57, 182
Anterior, 182
Anterior (position), 60
Antero, 5, 55, 60, 182
Anti, 57, 182
Append, 117, 121, 182
Archy, 95, 182
Arteri(o), 11, 115, 120, 182
Arthr(o), 11, 115, 120, 182
Astro, 14
Ate, 90, 182
Atric(s), 35, 182
Auto, 14, 59, 182
Autopsy, 20

Bacteriologist, 26
Bacteriology, 26
Basic system, 21
Bat, 14
Bi, 57, 182
Bilateral, 182
Bio, 20, 26, 59, 182
Biochemical genetics, 29
Biochemist, 26
Biochemistry, 26
Biological structure, 20
Biologist, 26, 27
Biology, 19, 20, 26, 59

Blephar(o), 118, 182
Board, 25
Board certification, 25
Board-certified, 25
Brady, 6, 57, 182
Bronch(o), 117, 121, 182
Brunne, 58, 182

Carcin(o), 119, 182
Card(i, io), 2, 4, 17, 21, 55, 115, 120, 182
Cardiologist, 21, 25, 27, 35
Cardiology, 2, 25, 27
Cardiovascular disease, 21, 27
Cardiovascular pharmacology, 25
Cardiovascular surgeon, 21, 27
Cardiovascular surgery, 27
Cardiovascular system, 21, 24
Caudal, 60, 182
Cavity, 60, 116, 182
Cele, 16, 90, 182
Cells, 20
Centesis, 94, 182
Centi, 13
Cephal(o), 8, 11, 60, 115, 120, 182
Cephalad, 60, 182
Chil(o), 8, 118, 182

Chlor(o), 2, 58, 182
Cholecyst(o), 117, 121, 182
Choledoch(o), 117, 121, 182
Chondr(o), 116, 120, 182
Chro, Chrom(a, o, at), 58, 119, 182
Cide, 95, 182
Cili(a, o), 118, 182
Circulatory system, 21, 24
Cirrh(o), 58, 182
Cise, 94, 182
Cle, 94, 183
Clinical epidemiologist, 27
Clinical genetics, 29
Clinical pathology, 34
Clinical pharmacology, 35, 36
Clinical pharmacy, 35
Coccyx, 116, 120
Col(o), 117, 121, 183
College of certification, 25
Colo-rectal surgery, 37
Colp(o), 117, 121, 183
Colpos, 118, 183
Comparative pathology, 34
Corp(o, us), 59, 118, 183
Cost(o), 63, 116, 120, 183
Crani(a, o), 17, 60, 117, 121, 183
Cranial, 60, 183
Cranium, 17
Cry(o), 119, 183
Crypt, 14, 55, 183
Cule, 94, 183
Cut(i), 8, 117, 121, 183
Cutane, 117, 121, 183
Cyan(o), 58, 183
Cyst(o), 116, 119, 120, 183
Cyt(o), 95, 118, 183
Cyte, 95, 118, 183
Cytologists, 22

De, 57, 183
Demi, 27
Dent(i, o), 8, 117, 121, 183
Derm(a, at), 13, 27, 117, 121, 183
Dermatologist, 22, 27
Dermatology, 27
Descriptive psychiatry, 37
Desis, 94, 183

Dextro, 8, 56, 183
Di, 57, 183
Dia, 14, 56, 183
Diabetes endocrinology, 27
Diagnostic and therapeutic (clinical) radiologist, 38
Digestive system, 21, 24
Dipl(o), 57, 183
Diplomate, 25
Distal, 3, 60, 117, 183
Doch(o), 118, 183
Dolicho, 59, 183
Dont, 117, 121, 183
Dorsal, 60, 66, 183
Dorsal lithotomy position, 65
Dorsal position, 64
Dorsal recumbent position, 64
Duct, 90, 183
Du(o), 58, 183
Dynamic psychiatry, 37
Dyne, 90, 184
Dynia, 90, 184
Dys, 8, 59, 184

Ec, 56, 91, 184
Ecta, 94, 184
Ectasis, 94, 184
Ecto, 56, 184
Ectomy, 94, 184
Ectop(y), 91, 184
Ectopic, 91, 184
Embryo, 20
Embryology, 19, 20
Emergency room physician, 27, 31
Emesis, 91, 184
Emia, 3, 184
Encephal(o), 11, 116, 120, 184
Endo, 56, 184
Endocrine system, 21, 24, 27
Endocrinologist, 23, 27, 38
Endocrinology, 21, 22, 27, 38
Ens, 91, 184
Enter(o), 10, 28, 117, 121, 184
Epi, 27, 56, 184
Epidemiologist, 27, 37
Epidemiology, 27, 31, 38
Epigastric region, 62
Erythro, 8, 59, 184

Eso, 56, 184
Esophag(o), 117, 121, 184
Esthes(ia), 2, 26, 94, 184
Etio, 8, 59, 184
Eu, 16, 58, 59, 184
Eum, 91, 184
Ex, 8, 56, 60, 184
Experimental pathology, 34
External, 37, 56, 60, 184
Extra, 56, 184

Family doctors, 28
Family practice, 26, 28, 29, 31, 36
Febr(o), 59, 184
Fellow, 25
Female reproductive system, 23
Femoral region, 62
Fetus, 20
Fibr(o), 118, 184
Five special senses, 22, 24
Flash cards, 4
Forensic (legal) pathology, 34
Form, 91, 184
Fowler, 184
Fowler position, 66
Ful, 91, 184

Gastr(o), 9, 21, 28, 117, 119, 121, 184
Gastroenterologist, 21, 28, 37
Gastroenterology, 28, 37
Gastrointestinal system, 21, 24
Gen(e, ic), 29, 91, 184
General practice, 28, 31, 36
General practitioner, 28, 36
Geneticist, 29
Genetics, 29
Genito, 21
Genitourinary system, 21, 23, 24, 39, 40
Geri, 29
Geriatrician, 29
Geriatrics, 29
Gerontology, 29
GIFT, 38
Glob(o), 119, 184
Gloss(o), 117, 121, 185
Gluc(o), 59, 185

Glyc(o), 59, 185
Gonads, 23
Gram, 91, 185
Graph, 13, 14, 90, 91, 185
Gyn(e, ec, eco), 23, 29, 60, 117, 185
Gynecologist, 23, 29, 33
Gynecology, 16, 25, 26, 29

Hem(a, o), 118, 119, 185
Hemat(o), 30, 118, 119, 185
Hematologist, 22, 30
Hematology, 30
Hemi, 56, 58, 185
Hepa(t, to), 117, 121, 185
Hernio, 185
Hetero, 5, 58
Hex(a), 58
Hist(o), 20, 118, 185
Histologist, 30
Homo, 3, 91
Hormones, 21
Hospice medicine, 30
Hypo, 5, 58, 185
Hypogastric region, 62
Hyster(o), 9, 117, 121, 185

Ia, 2, 17, 26, 55, 91, 185
Iasis, 91, 185
Ic, 2, 91, 185
Icle, 94, 185
Id, 91, 185
Ile(o), 9, 117, 121, 185
Ileum, 3, 18, 117
Ili(o), 9, 10, 116, 120, 185
Immuno-allergy, 26, 30, 31
Immunologist, 26, 30
Immunology, 26, 30
Industrial medicine, 31, 33
Infectious disease, 28, 31, 38
Inferior, 60, 185
Infra, 56, 185
Ino, 185
Integumentary, 24
Integumentary system, 22
Inter, 6, 56, 185
Intern, 31
Internal, 4, 31, 60, 185
Internal medicine, 28

Internist, 25, 31, 36
Internship, 25
Intra, 5, 56, 185
Ipsi, 56, 185
Ism, 91, 185
Ist, 13, 95, 185
Itis, 91, 185
Ium, 94, 185
IVF, 38
Ize, 94, 185

Kerat(o), 118, 119, 186
Kine(sis), 39, 186
Knee-chest position, 65, 186

Lapar(o), 5, 9, 116, 120, 186
Laryngo, 32, 34
Laryngologist, 32, 34
Laryngology, 32
Lateral, 3, 56, 58, 60, 183, 186
Lateral (position), 66, 186
Latero, 3, 56, 60, 186
Left hypochondriac region, 62
Left iliac region, 62
Left inguinal region, 62
Left lumbar region, 62
Lepsy, 91, 186
Lepto, 5, 59, 186
Leuc(o), 59, 186
Leuk(o), 59, 186
Levo, 56, 186
Lingu(o), 8, 117, 121, 186
Lip(o), 59, 60, 119, 180, 186
Lith(o), 95, 119, 186
Logy, 26, 91, 186
Lower right rectus incision, 64
Luna, 14
Lute, 59, 186
Lymph, 22
Lymphatic system, 22, 24
Lyse, 186
Lysis, 94, 186
Lytic, 94, 186

Macro, 59, 186
Magna, 2
Mal, 60, 186
Malacia, 91, 186
Male reproduction, 21

Male reproductive system, 23
Mast(o), 117, 121, 186
Maxillo, 32
Maxillofacial surgery, 32, 33
McBurney's incision, 64
Medial, 61, 186
Medicine, 25, 26, 28, 29, 31, 36
Medio, 5, 56, 186
Mega, 1, 5, 59, 186
Megaly, 94, 186
Melan, 59, 186
Meninges, 118, 186
Men(o), 119, 186
Mes(o), 56, 187
Meter, 14, 187
Metr(o), 9, 117, 121, 187
Metry, 14, 91, 187
Micro, 13, 59, 187
Microbiologist, 32
Microbiology, 32
Midline, 61, 186, 187
Midline incision, 63
Mid-rectus incision, 63
Mit, 92, 187
Mobile, 14
Mono, 58, 187
Morbid, 187
Muc(o), 119, 187
Multi, 58, 187
Muscular system, 22, 23, 24
Musculoskeletal system, 22, 23, 24
My(o), 116, 120, 187
Myc(o), 8, 119, 187
Myel(o), 116, 120, 187
Myo, 115, 116, 187
Myring(o), 118, 187

Narc, 5, 60, 187
Nas(o), 11, 39, 116, 120, 187
Nat, 14
Naut, 14
Necro, 5, 60, 187
Necropsy, 20
Neo, 57, 60, 187
Neonate, 35
Neonatology, 35
Nephr(o), 11, 32, 116, 120, 187
Nephrologist, 22, 32

Nephrology, 32, 40
Nervous system, 22, 23, 24
Neur(o), 11, 32, 115, 116, 120, 187
Neurological surgeons, 23
Neurological surgery, 32
Neurologist, 23, 32
Neurology, 32
Neurosurgeon, 32
Noct, 60, 187
Nost, 187
Nox, 60, 187
Nox(i), 60, 187
Nuclear medicine, 32, 38

Obstetri, 33, 187
Obstetrician, 33
Obstetrics, 25, 26, 29, 33, 38
Occupational medicine, 33
Ocul(o), 117, 121, 187
Oda, 92, 187
Odes, 92, 187
Oid, 92, 187
Ola, 94, 187
Ole, 94, 187
Olig(o), 119, 187
Ology, 2, 20, 92, 187
Oma, 92, 187
Onco(s), 33, 92, 118, 119, 187
Oncologist, 22, 32, 33, 35, 38, 95
Oncology, 33, 38
Onych(ia, o), 118, 187, 188
Oophor(o), 117, 121, 188
Op(t, tic), 118, 188
Ophthalm(o), 10, 33, 117, 121, 188
Ophthalmologist, 33
Ophthalmology, 23, 33
Opisth(o), 56, 188
Opt, 118
Optic, 118, 188
Or(o, a, i), 8, 116, 118, 120, 188
Oral pathology, 35
Oral surgeon, 33
Oral surgery, 32, 33
Orch(i, o, id), 116, 120, 188
Organs, 3, 4, 20, 21, 23
Or(i, o), 116, 188
Orth(o), 5, 33, 56, 188
Orthopedic surgeon, 33

Orthopedic surgery, 33
Orthopedics, 22, 26, 33, 36, 39
Orthopedist(s), 23, 33, 36, 39
Os, 92, 95, 188
Osis, 92, 188
Oste(o), 115, 116, 120, 188
Ostomy, 95
Ot(o), 10, 34, 117, 121, 188
Otic, 10, 118, 188
Otologist, 23, 34
Otology, 34
Otomy, 95, 188
Otorhinolaryngologist, 23, 32, 34
Otorhinolaryngology, 24, 34, 39
Ous, 92, 188
Ova, 23
Ovum, 20

Pain management, 34
Pan, 5, 58, 188
Pancreas, 117, 121
Para, 56, 188
Paramedian incision, 64
Parietal, 61, 188
Parous, 92, 188
Partum, 2, 92, 188
Pathogens, 22
Pathologist, 34
Pathology, 19, 20, 34, 60
Path(o, y), 20, 60, 92, 188
Ped (Greek), 95, 188
Ped (Latin), 13, 33, 95, 118, 188
Pedi(a), 35, 95, 188
Pediatric specialties, 25
Pediatrician, 35
Pediatrics, 35
Penia, 92, 188
Pep(s), 119, 188
Peri, 14, 56, 188
Peripheral, 61, 188
Pexy, 95, 188
Phag(o), 92, 188
Pharmac, 35
Pharmacist, 35
Pharmacologist, 35
Pharmacology, 35
Pharmacy, 35
Pharyng(o), 117, 121, 188
Phasia, 92, 188
Phleb(o), 11, 115, 116, 120, 188

Phobia, 92, 188
Phon(e, o), 3, 13
Phoresis, 92, 188
Phyll, 92, 189
Physic, 36
Physical medicine and rehabilitation, 33, 36, 39
Physical therapist, 36
Physio, 20
Physiology, 19, 20
Plasm, 92, 189
Plas(t, ty), 36, 92, 95, 189
Plastic surgeon, 36
Plastic surgery, 36
Pleur(a, o), 116, 118, 120, 189
Pnea, 92, 189
Pneum(o), 117, 121, 189
Pod, 95, 118, 189
Poie, 119, 189
Poly, 58, 189
Positions for surgery and examination, 64
Post, 2, 56, 57, 189
Posterior, 61, 189
Postero, 56, 61, 189
Pre, 14, 55, 56, 57, 189
Prenatal pediatrics, 35
Primary care physician, 28, 31, 36
Proct(o), 37, 117, 121, 189
Proctologist, 21, 37
Proctology, 28, 37
Prone, 61
Prone position, 66, 189
Prostat(o), 116, 120, 189
Proximal, 61, 189
Pseudo, 189
Psychiatrist, 37
Psychiatry, 37
Psychiatry, child and adolescent, 37
Psychology, 37
Ptosis, 3, 92, 189
Ptysis, 3, 92, 189
Public health, 28, 31, 37
Pulmo, 38
Pulmonary disease, 23, 38
Purpur, 59, 189
Pyel(o), 8, 116, 120, 189
Pyo, 5, 60, 189

Pyr(o), 60, 189

Quadr(o, u), 58, 189
Quadrants, 61

Rachi(a, o), 116, 120, 189
Rachis, 116, 119, 120
Radiation oncologist, 32, 38
Radio, 38
Radiologist, 32
Radiology, 32, 38
Re, 23
Reconstructive surgery, 36
Rehabilitative medicine, 36
Ren(i, o), 11, 116, 120, 189
Renal, 11, 119, 189
Reproductive endocrinologist, 23
Reproductive endocrinology, 21,
    22, 27, 29, 33, 38
Reproductive system, 22, 23, 24
Residency, 25
Resident, 31
Respiratory system, 23, 24
Retro, 56, 189
Rheumatologist, 38
Rheumatology, 22, 38
Rhin(o), 34, 39, 116, 120, 189
Rhinologist, 34, 39
Rhinology, 39
Right hypochondriac region, 62
Right iliac region, 62
Right inguinal region, 62
Right lumbar region, 62
Rrhage, 92, 189
Rrhagia, 92, 189
Rrhaphy, 95, 189
Rrhea, 92, 189
Rrhexis, 93, 189

Sacr(o), 116, 120, 190
Salping(o), 10, 118, 121, 188
Schiz(o), 190
Scler(o), 93, 190
Scope, 13, 14. 93, 190
Scopy, 93, 190
Semi, 5, 58, 190
Sep(t), 2, 190
Sex(i), 58, 190
Sims position, 66, 190

Sis, 93, 190
Skeletal system, 22, 23, 24
Skin system, 22, 24
Sociologist, 39
Sociology, 39
Sophy, 95, 190
Spasm, 93, 190
Specul(o), 190
Sperm, 20, 22, 23
Spire, 23, 93, 190
Splen(o), 118, 121, 190
Sports medicine, 33, 39
Stalsis, 93, 190
Stasis, 93, 190
Stat, 190
Stat (abbr.), 190
Static, 190
Staxis, 93, 190
Sten(o), 14, 116, 190
Stern(o), 116, 120, 190
Stom(a), 93, 190
Stomach, 119
Sub, 1, 56, 63, 190
Subcostal incision, 63
Sui, 60, 190
Super, 56, 190
Superior, 61, 190
Supine, 61, 65, 66, 187, 190
Supine position, 64
Supra, 56, 64, 190
Suprapubic incision, 64
Suprapubic region, 62
Surgeons, 21, 22
Surgery, 7, 25, 28, 39
Surgical pathology, 35
Systems, 3, 20, 21

Tach(o, y), 5, 14, 55, 58, 190
Tax(o), 93, 190
Taxi, 93
Taxi(s), 13, 93, 190
Tele, 1, 13, 14, 57, 190
Tetra, 58, 190
Therm, 190
Thorac(o), 39, 116, 120, 190
Thoracic surgeon, 21, 39
Thromb(o), 8, 119, 191
Thyr(o), 116, 120, 191
Tic, 14, 93, 188, 191

Tinea, 7, 8, 191
Tissue and cytological pathology,
    35
Tissues, 20
Tomy, 19, 95, 191
Topy, 91, 191
Trache(o), 118, 121, 191
Trans, 13, 57, 191
Transverse incision, 64
Trendelenberg position, 65, 191
Tri, 58, 191
Trophy, 36, 93, 191
Tropic, 93, 191
Tropism, 93, 191

Ule, 94, 191
Ulous, 93, 191
Ulum, 94, 191
Ulus, 94, 191
Umbilical region, 62
Umbilicus, 64
Uni, 58, 191
Upper right rectus incision, 63
Ur(e, ia, in, o), 21, 39, 93, 191
Ureter(o), 116, 120, 191
Urological surgery/urological sur-
    geon, 39
Urologist, 22, 23, 39
Urology, 32, 38, 39
Urticaria, 26, 191
Uter(o), 35, 118, 121, 191

Vari, 6, 57, 58, 191
Vascular surgeon, 40
Vascular surgeons, 21
Vascular surgery, 40
Vas(o), 8, 21, 27, 40, 119, 191
Ventral, 61, 191
Visceral, 61, 191
Vox, 2

Womb, 9, 118, 121

Xantho, 59, 191
Xero, 191

ZIFT, 38